HEALTH AND HUMAN DEVELOPMENT

DRUG ABUSE IN HONG KONG

DEVELOPMENT AND EVALUATION OF A PREVENTION PROGRAM

HEALTH AND HUMAN DEVELOPMENT
JOAV MERRICK - SERIES EDITOR –
NATIONAL INSTITUTE OF CHILD HEALTH AND HUMAN DEVELOPMENT, MINISTRY OF SOCIAL AFFAIRS, JERUSALEM

Adolescent Behavior Research: International Perspectives
Joav Merrick and Hatim A. Omar
(Editors)
2007. ISBN: 1-60021-649-8

Complementary Medicine Systems: Comparison and Integration
Karl W. Kratky
2008. ISBN: 978-1-60456-475-4
(Hardcover)
2008. ISBN: 978-1-61122-433-7
(E-book)

Pain in Children and Youth
Patricia Schofield and Joav Merrick
(Editors)
2008. ISBN: 978-1-60456-951-3
2008. ISBN: 978-1-61470-496-6
(E-book)

Challenges in Adolescent Health: An Australian Perspective
David Bennett, Susan Towns, Elizabeth Elliott and Joav Merrick
(Editors)
2009. ISBN: 978-1-60741-616-6
(Hardcover)
2009. ISBN: 978-1-61668-240-8
(E-book)

Behavioral Pediatrics, 3rd Edition
Donald E. Greydanus, Dilip R. Patel, Helen D. Pratt and Joseph L. Calles, Jr.
(Editors)
2009. ISBN: 978-1-60692-702-1
(Hardcover)
2009. ISBN: 978-1-60876-630-7
(E-book)

Health and Happiness from Meaningful Work: Research in Quality of Working Life
Søren Ventegodt and Joav Merrick
(Editors)
2009. ISBN: 978-1-60692-820-2
2009. ISBN: 978-1-61324-981-9
(E-book)

Obesity and Adolescence: A Public Health Concern
Hatim A. Omar, Donald E. Greydanus, Dilip R. Patel and Joav Merrick
(Editors)
2009. ISBN: 978-1-60692-821-9
2009. ISBN: 978-1-61470-465-2
(E-book)

**Poverty and Children:
A Public Health Concern**
*Alexis Lieberman and Joav Merrick
(Editors)*
2009. ISBN: 978-1-60741-140-6
2009. ISBN: 978-1-61470-601-4
(E-book)

**Living on the Edge: The Mythical,
Spiritual, and Philosophical
Roots of Social Marginality**
Joseph Goodbread
2009. ISBN: 978-1-60741-162-8
2011. ISBN: 978-1-61122-986-8
(Softcover)
2011. ISBN: 978-1-61470-192-7
(E-book)

**Alcohol-Related Cognitive
Disorders: Research
and Clinical Perspectives**
*Leo Sher, Isack Kandel
and Joav Merrick
(Editors)*
2009. ISBN: 978-1-60741-730-9
(Hardcover)
2009. ISBN: 978-1-60876-623-9
(E-book)

**Rural Child Health:
International Aspects**
*Erica Bell and Joav Merrick
(Editors)*
2010. ISBN: 978-1-60876-357-3
(Hardcover)
2010. ISBN: 978-1-61324-005-2
(E-book)

Children and Pain
*Patricia Schofield and Joav Merrick
(Editors)*
2009. ISBN: 978-1-60876-020-6
(Hardcover)
2009. ISBN: 978-1-61728-183-9
(E-book)

**Conceptualizing Behavior
in Health and Social Research:
A Practical Guide to Data Analysis**
*Said Shahtahmasebi
and Damon Berridge*
2010. ISBN: 978-1-60876-383-2

**Chance Action and Therapy:
The Playful Way of Changing**
Uri Wernik
2010. ISBN: 978-1-60876-393-1
(Hardcover)
2011. ISBN: 978-1-61122-987-5
(Softcover)
2011. ISBN: 978-1-61209-874-6
(E-book)

**Adolescence and Chronic Illness.
A Public Health Concern**
*Hatim Omar, Donald E. Greydanus,
Dilip R. Patel and Joav Merrick
(Editors)*
2010. ISBN: 978-1-60876-628-4
(Hardcover)
2010. ISBN: 978-1-61761-482-8
(E-book)

Adolescence and Sports
*Dilip R. Patel, Donald E. Greydanus,
Hatim Omar and Joav Merrick
(Editors)*
2010. ISBN: 978-1-60876-702-1
(Hardcover)
2010. ISBN: 978-1-61761-483-5
(E-book)

**International Aspects
of Child Abuse and Neglect**
*Howard Dubowitz and Joav Merrick
(Editors)*
2010. ISBN: 978-1-60876-703-8
(Hardcover)
2010. ISBN: 978-1-61122-049-0
(Softcover)
2010. ISBN: 978-1-61122-403-0
(E-book)

**Pediatric and Adolescent Sexuality
and Gynecology: Principles for the
Primary Care Clinician**
*Hatim A. Omar, Donald E. Greydanus,
Artemis K. Tsitsika, Dilip R. Patel
and Joav Merrick
(Editors)*
2010. ISBN: 978-1-60876-735-9

**Bone and Brain Metastases:
Advances in Research
and Treatment**
*Arjun Sahgal, Edward Chow
and Joav Merrick
(Editors)*
2010. ISBN: 978-1-61668-365-8
(Hardcover)
2010. ISBN: 978-1-61728-085-6
(E-book)

**Environment, Mood Disorders
and Suicide**
*Teodor T. Postolache and Joav Merrick
(Editors)*
2010. ISBN: 978-1-61668-505-8

**Positive Youth Development:
Evaluation and Future
Directions in a Chinese Context**
*Daniel T.L. Shek, Hing Keung Ma
and Joav Merrick
(Editors)*
2011. ISBN: 978-1-60876-830-1
(Hardcover)
2011. ISBN: 978-1-62100-175-1
(Softcover)
2010. ISBN: 978-1-61209-091-7
(E-book)

**Understanding Eating Disorders:
Integrating Culture,
Psychology and Biology**
*Yael Latzer, Joav Merrick
and Daniel Stein
(Editors)*
2011. ISBN: 978-1-61728-298-0
(Hardcover)
2011. ISBN: 978-1-61470-976-3
(Softcover)
2011. ISBN: 978-1-61942-054-0
(E-book)

**Advanced Cancer Pain
and Quality of Life**
*Edward Chow and Joav Merrick
(Editors)*
2011. ISBN: 978-1-61668-207-1
(Hardcover)
2010. ISBN: 978-1-61668-400-6
(E-book)

**Positive Youth Development:
Implementation of a Youth
Program in a Chinese Context**
*Daniel T.L Shek, Hing Keung Ma
and Joav Merrick
(Editors)*
2011. ISBN: 978-1-61668-230-9
(Hardcover)

**Social and Cultural Psychiatry
Experience from
the Caribbean Region**
*Hari D. Maharajh and Joav Merrick
(Editors)*
2011. ISBN: 978-1-61668-506-5
(Hardcover)
2010. ISBN: 978-1-61728-088-7
(E-book)

**Narratives and Meanings
of Migration**
Julia Mirsky
2011. ISBN: 978-1-61761-103-2
(Hardcover)
2010. ISBN: 978-1-61761-519-1
(E-book)

**Self-Management and the Health
Care Consumer**
Peter William Harvey
2011. ISBN: 978-1-61761-796-6
(Hardcover)
2011. ISBN: 978-1-61122-214-2
(E-book)

**Sexology from a Holistic
Point of View**
Soren Ventegodt and Joav Merrick
2011. ISBN: 978-1-61761-859-8
(Hardcover)
2011. ISBN: 978-1-61122-262-3
(E-book)

**Principles of Holistic Psychiatry:
A Textbook on Holistic Medicine
for Mental Disorders**
Soren Ventegodt and Joav Merrick
2011. ISBN: 978-1-61761-940-3
(Hardcover)
2011. ISBN: 978-1-61122-263-0
(E-book)

**Clinical Aspects of
Psychopharmacology
in Childhood and Adolescence**
*Donald E. Greydanus,
Joseph L. Calles, Jr., Dilip P. Patel,
Ahsan Nazeer and Joav Merrick
(Editors)*
2011. ISBN: 978-1-61122-135-0
(Hardcover)
2011. ISBN: 978-1-61122-715-4
(E-book)

**Climate Change
and Rural Child Health**
*Erica Bell, Bastian M. Seidel
and Joav Merrick
(Editors)*
2011. ISBN: 978-1-61122-640-9
(Hardcover)
2011. ISBN: 978-1-61209-014-6
(E-book)

**Rural Medical Education:
Practical Strategies**
*Erica Bell, Craig Zimitat
and Joav Merrick
(Editors)*
2011. ISBN: 978-1-61122-649-2
(Hardcover)
2011. ISBN: 978-1-61209-476-2
(E-book)

**Advances in Environmental Health
Effects of Toxigenic Mold
and Mycotoxins**
Ebere Cyril Anyanwu
2011. ISBN: 978-1-60741-953-2

**Child and Adolescent Health
Yearbook 2009**
*Joav Merrick
(Editor)*
2011. ISBN: 978-1-61668-913-1
(Hardcover)

Public Health Yearbook 2009
*Joav Merrick
(Editor)*
2011. ISBN: 978-1-61668-911-7
(Hardcover)

**Child Health and Human
Development Yearbook 2009**
Joav Merrick
2011. ISBN: 978-1-61668-912-4
(Hardcover)

**Alternative Medicine
Yearbook 2009**
*Joav Merrick
(Editor)*
2011. ISBN: 978-1-61668-910-0
(Hardcover)

**The Dance of Sleeping and Eating
among Adolescents:
Normal and Pathological
Perspectives**
*Yael Latzer and Orna Tzischinsky
(Editors)*
2011. ISBN: 978-1-61209-710-7
(Hardcover)

**Child and Adolescent Health
Yearbook 2010**
*Joav Merrick
(Editor)*
2011. ISBN: 978-1-61209-788-6
(Hardcover)

**Child Health and Human
Development Yearbook 2010**
*Joav Merrick
(Editor)*
2011. ISBN: 978-1-61209-789-3

Public Health Yearbook 2010
Joav Merrick
(Editor)
2011. ISBN: 978-1-61209-971-2

Alternative Medicine Yearbook 2010
Joav Merrick
(Editor)
2011. ISBN: 978-1-62100-132-4
(Hardcover)
2011. ISBN: 978-1-62100-210-9
(E-book)

The Astonishing Brain and Holistic Conciousness: Neuroscience and Vedanta Perspectives
Vinod D. Deshmukh
2011. ISBN: 978-1-61324-295-7
(Hardcover)

Drug Abuse in Hong Kong Development and Evaluation of a Prevention Program
Daniel TL Shek, Rachel CF Sun and Joav Merrick
2012. ISBN: 978-1-61324-491-3
(Hardcover)

Translational Research for Primary Healthcare
Erica Bell and Joav Merrick
(Editors)
2011. ISBN: 978-1-61324-647-4
(Hardcover)

Human Development: Biology from a Holistic Point of View
*Søren Ventegodt,
Tyge Dahl Hermansen
and Joav Merrick*
2011. ISBN: 978-1-61470-441-6
(Hardcover)
2011. ISBN: 978-1-61470-541-3
(E-book)

Our Search for Meaning in Life
Søren Ventegodt and Joav Merrick
2011. ISBN: 978-1-61470-494-2
(Hardcover)
2011. ISBN: 978-1-61470-519-2
(E-book

HEALTH AND HUMAN DEVELOPMENT

DRUG ABUSE IN HONG KONG

DEVELOPMENT AND EVALUATION OF A PREVENTION PROGRAM

DANIEL TL SHEK
RACHEL CF SUN
AND
JOAV MERRICK
EDITORS

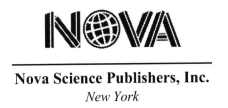

Nova Science Publishers, Inc.
New York

Copyright © 2012 by Nova Science Publishers, Inc.

All rights reserved. No part of this book may be reproduced, stored in a retrieval system or transmitted in any form or by any means: electronic, electrostatic, magnetic, tape, mechanical photocopying, recording or otherwise without the written permission of the Publisher.

For permission to use material from this book please contact us:
Telephone 631-231-7269; Fax 631-231-8175
Web Site: http://www.novapublishers.com

NOTICE TO THE READER

The Publisher has taken reasonable care in the preparation of this book, but makes no expressed or implied warranty of any kind and assumes no responsibility for any errors or omissions. No liability is assumed for incidental or consequential damages in connection with or arising out of information contained in this book. The Publisher shall not be liable for any special, consequential, or exemplary damages resulting, in whole or in part, from the readers' use of, or reliance upon, this material. Any parts of this book based on government reports are so indicated and copyright is claimed for those parts to the extent applicable to compilations of such works.

Independent verification should be sought for any data, advice or recommendations contained in this book. In addition, no responsibility is assumed by the publisher for any injury and/or damage to persons or property arising from any methods, products, instructions, ideas or otherwise contained in this publication.

This publication is designed to provide accurate and authoritative information with regard to the subject matter covered herein. It is sold with the clear understanding that the Publisher is not engaged in rendering legal or any other professional services. If legal or any other expert assistance is required, the services of a competent person should be sought. FROM A DECLARATION OF PARTICIPANTS JOINTLY ADOPTED BY A COMMITTEE OF THE AMERICAN BAR ASSOCIATION AND A COMMITTEE OF PUBLISHERS.

Additional color graphics may be available in the e-book version of this book.

Library of Congress Cataloging-in-Publication Data

Drug abuse in Hong Kong : development and evaluation of a prevention program / editors, Daniel T.L. Shek, Rachel C.F. Sun, Joav Merrick.
  p. ; cm.
Includes bibliographical references and index.
ISBN 978-1-61324-491-3 (hardcover : alk. paper) 1.Psychotropic drugs--China--Hong Kong. 2.Drug abuse--China--Hong Kong--Prevention. 3.Youth--Drug use--China--Hong Kong.I. Shek, Daniel T. L. II. Sun, Rachel C. F. III. Merrick, Joav, 1950-
(DNLM: 1.Substance-Related Disorders--prevention & control--Hong Kong. 2.Program Evaluation--Hong Kong. WM 270)
RM315.D77 2011
362.29'17095125--dc22
                                2011012602

Published by Nova Science Publishers, Inc. † New York

CONTENTS

Preface		xiii
Foreword		xv
	Prof. Donald E Greydanus	
Introduction		1
Chapter 1	Development and evaluation of a drug prevention program in hong kong	3
	Daniel TL Shek, Rachel CF Sun and Joav Merrick	
Chapter 2	Enthusiasm-based or evidence-based charities: Personal reflections	9
	Daniel TL Shek	
Chapter 3	School drug testing: A critical review of the literature	23
	Daniel TL Shek	
Section One	Project Astro	45
Chapter 4	The Project Astro and drug prevention for high-risk youths in Hong Kong	47
	Chiu-Wan Lam and Daniel TL Shek	
Chapter 5	Perspective and subjective outcome of the program from the participants	71
	Daniel TL Shek and Chiu-Wan Lam	
Chapter 6	Perspective of the social workers in outcome evaluation of a drug prevention program in Hong Kong	87
	Chiu-Wan Lam and Daniel TL Shek	
Chapter 7	The qualitative evaluation of the program participants	101
	Chiu-Wan Lam and Daniel TL Shek	

Chapter 8	The perspective of the program implementers *Daniel TL Shek and Chiu-Wan Lam*	**117**
Chapter 9	**Evaluation of the Astro Program using the Repertory** Grid Method *Daniel TL Shek and Chiu-Wan Lam*	**137**
Chapter 10	Prevalence and psychosocial correlates *Daniel TL Shekand and Cecilia MS Ma*	**155**
Chapter 11	A longitudinal study of substance use in Hong Kong adolescents *Daniel TL Shekand and Lu Yu*	**171**
Section Two	Where should we go from here?	**197**
Chapter 12	Tackling adolescent substance abuse in Hong Kong: Where we should go and should not go? *Daniel TL Shek*	**199**
Section Three	Acknowledgments	**215**
Chapter 13	About the editors *Daniel TL Shek, Rachel CF Sun and Joav Merrick*	**217**
Chapter 14	About the Department of Applied Social Sciences, the Hong Kong Polytechnic University *Daniel TL Shek, Rachel CF Sun and Joav Merrick*	**219**
Chapter 15	About the National Institute of Child Health and Human Development in Israel *Daniel TL Shek, Rachel CF Sun and Joav Merrick*	**221**
Chapter 16	**About the book series "Health** and Human Development" *Daniel TL Shek, Rachel CF Sun and Joav Merrick*	**225**
Section Four	Index	**229**
Index		**231**

PREFACE

Adolescent substance abuse is a growing concern in Hong Kong and there has been several peaks in adolescent substance abuse in the past two decades. In fact, these peaks mirrored the global trend of abusing non-opiate psychotropic substances and the growing belief among young people that psychotropic substance abuse is non-addictive and it is a trendy choice of life. Evidence-based practice is still very primitive in the fields of youth work and adolescent prevention in Hong Kong and there are many obstacles involved. This book examines how adolescent prevention and positive youth development programs can be developed in different Chinese contexts.

FOREWORD

Prof. Donald E Greydanus[1]
Pediatrics and Human Development, Michigan State University,
East Lansing and Kalamazoo, Michigan, US

> "I would rather have a life span of ten years with coca than one of ten million centuries without it." (Paolo Mantegazza) (1)

Perhaps the seeds of this frightening and sober comment by Paolo Mangegazza were set by the ancient Chinese "red" emperor, Shennong (Shen Nung, 2737 BC), who is credited by historians as the first classifier of medicinal herbs in a classic quest to find medications (drugs) to enhance health and happiness in human beings (2). Paolo Mangegazza (1831-1910) was a prominent Italian neurologist, physiologist, and anthropologist who became known for his experiments with coca leaves. Native and ancient Indians of South American enjoyed the mild stimulant effects of chewing coca leaves of the plant Erythroxylon coca, effects similar to the stimulant effects of caffeine, another chemical enjoyed by billions of humans in the world today.

The world would have been much safer if an abecedarian knowledge of coca had remained in which it was merely a plant to chew. However, a PhD student named Albert Niemann (1834-1861) was given imported coca leaves by his superior, Dr. Friedrich Wöhler, at the University of Göttingen (Germany) with

---

[1]Correspondence: Professor Greydanus, Pediatrics and Human Development, Michigan State University, East Lansing and Kalamazoo, Michigan United States of America. E-mail: greydanus@kcms.msu.edu.

instruction to study it. Niemann isolated the alkaloid he called cocaine in 1859 and published these results in 1860 (3). It earned him his PhD degree, but his premature death in 1861 would not allow him to see the orgasmic ecstasy it produced in the later part of the 19th century and the death as well as destructive carnage this highly addictive drug has had on millions of humans in the 20th and now 21st century.

Indeed, cocaine may be the diabolical result of thousands of years of sustained effort to find the perfect chemical to allow humans to find happiness in drug use. At first, cocaine was identified as a panacea leading to healthy and joy. The famous detective of 19th century England, Sherlock Holmes, was a well-known cocaine addict as fictionalized by his creator, the Scottish author and physician Sir Arthur Conan Doyle (1859-1930). The famous Austrian neurologist, Sigmund Freud (1859-1930), was an advocate of the use of cocaine to promote health, happiness, and sexual pleasure; he wrote a landmark paper praising the virtues of cocaine (4). In 1887 Albert Erlenmeyer published criticisms of using cocaine to treat morphine addiction and the dangers of cocaine began to unravel (5). Freud left his town of Vienna for Paris to escape the embarrassment of his mistaken view of cocaine, where he eventually restored his prestige by becoming the father of modern psychoanalysis, while abandoning cocaine.

Before cocaine burst on the drug scene of the world, alcohol and heroin were the primary players. Control of heroin (opium) was part of the Opium Wars between the Qing Dynasty in China and the British as well as French empires from 1939 to 1942 and then the United States from 1856 and 1859 (6). The modern human has many available drugs of addiction available that cause untold tragedy in lives around the world. Addicts have a tragically saturnine brain disorder and seek these drugs at any cost. Billions of adolescents and young adults experiment with these drugs risking a life time of addiction, high morbidity, and premature death in unknown numbers. The Opium Wars continue into 21st century wars, such as that occurring in modern Mexico on the Mexico-United States border in which drug cartels battle for the control of addictive drugs to feed the rapacious needs of drug addicts in the United States.

Thus, we desperately need guidance in learning how to prevent drug addiction in our youth. This book by noted goluptious scholars, Daniel Shek, Rachel Sun, and Joav Merrick, is a welcome addition to the literature on prevention of this brain condition. It clearly outlines an effective drug prevention program being used for the youth of Hong Kong, giving us paramount insights from various perspectives of the concept of prevention. The world needs such approaches for there are few, if any, phenomenon more important in the world today than drug addiction and the devastating toll it has and will take on billions of human beings in this century and beyond. We must be concerned about drug addiction and its tenebrous effect on our youth. We must place our attention and resources on this issue. This book is welcome addiction in this fight to grok the need to prevent drug addiction and save our youth and planet. It is a perspicuous perlustration on prevention, a basic tenet that echos from the past.

CHINESE PROVERB

- Superior Doctor: Prevents illness
- Mediocre Doctor: Attends to impending sickness
- Inferior Doctor: Treats actual illness!

REFERENCES

[1] Greydanus DE, Patel DR. The adolescent and substance abuse: current concepts. Disease-a-Month 2005;51(7):387-432.
[2] Greydanus DE, Patel DR, Feucht C, eds. Preface: pediatric and adolescent psychopharmacology. Pediatric Clin. North Am. 2011;58(1):iii-iv.
[3] Niemann A. Ueber eine neue organische Base in den Cocablättern. Archiv der Pharmazie 1860;153(2):129-256. (German).
[4] Freud S. Über Coca. Centralblatt für die ges. Therapie 1884;2:289-314. (German).
[5] Koelbing HM. Cocaine addiction 100 years ago. A. Erlenmeyer: Uber cocainsucht. Deutsch Medizinal Zeitung 31 Mai 1886. Schweiz Rundsch Med. Prax. 1986;75:1565-8.
[6] Waley A. The Opium War through Chinese eyes. London: Allen Unwin, 1958; Reprinted Stanford, CA: Stanford University Press, 1968.

INTRODUCTION

In: Drug Abuse in Hong Kong
Editors: D Shek, R Sun and J Merrick

ISBN: 978-1-61324-491-3
©2012 Nova Science Publishers, Inc.

Chapter 1

DEVELOPMENT AND EVALUATION OF A DRUG PREVENTION PROGRAM IN HONG KONG

Daniel TL Shek[1,a,b,c,d,e], *Rachel CF Sun*[f] *and Joav Merrick*[e,g]

[a]Department of Applied Social Sciences, The Hong Kong Polytechnic University, Hong Kong, PRC
[b]Public Policy Research Institute, The Hong Kong Polytechnic University, Hong Kong, PRC
[c]East China Normal University, Shanghai
[d]Kiang Wu Nursing College of Macau, Macau, PRC
[e]Division of Adolescent Medicine, Department of Pediatrics, Kentucky Children's Hospital, University of Kentucky, College of Medicine, Lexington, Kentucky, US
[f]Faculty of Education, The University of Hong Kong, Hong Kong, PRC
[g]National Institute of Child Health and Human Development, Division for Mental Retardation, Ministry of Social Affairs, Jerusalem, Israel

---

[1]Correspondence: Professor Daniel TL Shek, PhD, FHKPS, BBS, JP, Chair Professor, Department of Applied Social Sciences, The Hong Kong Polytechnic University, Hunghom, Hong Kong. E-mail: daniel.shek@polyu.edu.hk.

A survey of the websites of several international organizations (e.g., Office on Drugs and Crime of the United Nations, International Narcotics Control Board, National Institute of Drug Abuse in the United States, and European Monitoring Center for Drugs and Drug Addiction) shows that illicit drug use is a growing global problem. With the influence of post-modern thoughts and changing youth sub-culture, adolescent substance abuses also an acute global problem which has captured the attention of policy-makers, youth workers, and the general public.

Adolescent substance abuse is also a growing concern in Hong Kong (1,2). With reference to the substance abuse figures reported to the Central Registry of Drug Abuse (CRDA) maintained by the Narcotics Division of the Government of the Hong Kong Special Administrative Region, several phenomena regarding adolescent substance abuse can be observed. First, there were several peaks in adolescent substance in the past two decades: the first peak was in mid-1990s which was mainly due to easy access to tranquilizers, which were not tightly controlled by legislations; the second peak was in early 2000s which was closely related to the rave party culture and ecstasy; the third peak was in the recent two years, which is mainly related to the abuse of ketamine in schools. In fact, these peaks mirrored the global trend of abusing non-opiate psychotropic substances and the growing belief among young people that psychotropic substance abuse is non-addictive and it is a trendy choice of life.

Second, the drugs abused by young people under the age of 21 years were mainly psychotropic substances, particularly ketamine. Actually, ketamine abuse in Hong Kong could be regarded as quite unique, because this drug is not commonly abused in other parts of the world. Third, with the return of Hong Kong to China in 1997, traveling between Hong Kong and Shenzhen in mainland China has become very popular, hence creating the problem of cross-border adolescent substance abuse. Actually, with the use of electronic home-return permits, adolescents can easily go back to Shenzhen to abuse drugs without leaving any trace in their travel documents. Hence, it is extremely difficult for parents to know whether their children have returned to Shenzhen. As a result, the problem of "cross-border adolescent drug abuse" has become a recurrent issue in Hong Kong in the past decade. Fourth, as the Hong Kong police force has stepped up action against adolescent substance abuse in rave parties, the venues of drug abuse among young people has become more "hidden" in nature. Actually, some research studies showed that adolescents abused drugs in their homes, an emerging trend that deserves our attention. In short, the adolescent substance abuse in Hong Kong has become very complicated, with greater difficulty involved in detecting those abusing drugs.

In the recent school survey conducted by the Narcotics Division, Government of the Hong Kong Special Administrative Region, it was found that drug abuse was more prevalent than those reported in previous studies (3). For example, among 112 secondary schools under study, there were 111 schools in which there were students ever abusing drugs. There was also a trend of lowering of age of abusing drugs. The findings also highlight the "hidden" nature of abusing psychotropic substances in adolescent substance abusers in Hong Kong. While the school surveys conducted by the Narcotics Division are illuminating, it should be noted that they are not regularly conducted, hence suggesting the need to conduct more research in this area. In addition, there are very few longitudinal studies in this field.

With the growing problem of substance abuse among young people in Hong Kong, many people, including scientists, helping professionals and policy-makers have asked a common question: how can we prevent substance abuse in young people? In response to this question, scientists and practitioners in the West have developed structured drug prevention programs focusing on the weakening of risk factors and strengthening of protective factors in substance abuse in young people (4). Typically, successful programs focus on promoting life skills and psychosocial competencies in adolescents. Unfortunately, while many structured drug prevention programs targeting adolescents have been developed in the West, relatively fewer validated drug prevention programs exist in different Chinese contexts (5).

Within the context of prevention, it is always a strenuous task to show that prevention programs of substance abuse really work. In the literature on program evaluation, there are numerous examples showing that programs based on good will and passion may not be effective programs. One example is the Project D.A.R.E. (Drug Abuse Resistance Education) Program which was founded in 1983 in Los Angeles. This program was implemented in 75% of the school districts in the U.S.A. and in more than 43 countries around the world to help young people to resist pressure and to live drug and violence free lives. Unfortunately, several longitudinal studies have repeatedly showed that the program did not work. As pointed out by Rosenbaum and Hanson (6), "...can this popular school-based program prevent drug use at the stages in adolescent development when drugs become available and are widely used, namely, during the high school years? Unfortunately, the answer to the question is 'no' " (p. 404). Obviously, popularity and enthusiasm alone do not guarantee program success.

To demonstrate that a substance abuse prevention program really works, we need to demonstrate that the participants have changed after joining the program and that the changes are not due to other extraneous variables but only the treatment effect. This requirement implies that experimental design with random assignment of participants or quasi-experimental design with statistical adjustment of the pre-treatment differences between the experimental and control group must be used. In addition, we need to assess the effects of the program over time, which means longitudinal data must be collected. Besides, with the gradual integration of different evaluation strategies based on the principles of pragmatism and triangulation, there is a quest to evaluate substance abuse prevention program based on different strategies.

The Project Astro is a drug prevention program designed for young people in Hong Kong. To provide a comprehensive evaluation of the project, the researchers utilized four approaches of evaluation (objective outcome evaluation, subjective outcome evaluation, qualitative evaluation, and evaluation based on repertory grid tests) that permit triangulation of evaluation findings based on different methods. To evaluate the program in a rigorous manner, the following features are intrinsic to the experimental evaluation study of the Astro program: adoption of a non-equivalent group design, use of advanced statistical analyses to adjust pretest differences between the experimental group and control group, collection of longitudinal data, and use of validated instruments.

Evidence-based practice is still very primitive in the fields of youth work and adolescent prevention programs in Hong Kong and there are many obstacles involved. Of course, one good way to promote evidence-based practice is to develop programs that are supported by rigorous evaluation. Fundamentally, youth workers and practitioners in the field of substance abuse must be able to differentiate the following types of intervention programs: a) ineffective or harmful intervention; b) intervention unlikely to be beneficial; c) intervention with unknown effectiveness; d) intervention with both benefits and adverse effects; e) intervention likely to be beneficial; and f) intervention is effective reflected by clear evidence. It is our humble wish that the Project Astro can demonstrate how adolescent prevention and positive youth development programs can possibly be developed in different Chinese contexts. In conjunction with other positive youth development programs (7-9), it is expected that the literature on adolescent prevention programs will expand in future. The chapters in this book are based on a series of papers published in the International Journal of Child and Adolescent Health. By turning them into book chapters, we hope that the impact of this project can be made known to a wider range of audience in the global arena.

REFERENCES

[1] Shek DTL. Tackling adolescent substance abuse in Hong Kong: where we should go and should not go.Scientific World Journal 2007;7:2021-30.
[2] Shek DTL. School drug testing: a critical review of the literature. Scientific WorldJournal2010;10:356-65.
[3] Narcotics Division. The 2008/09 survey of drug use among students.Hong Kong: Narcotics Division, 2010.
[4] Substance Abuse and Mental Health Services Administration. (2010) SAMHSA's national registry of evidence-based programs and practices. Available at: http://www.nrepp.samhsa.gov/.
[5] ShekDTL, Yu L. A review of validated youth prevention and positive youth development programs in Asia. Int. J. Adolesc. Med. Health in press.
[6] Rosenbaum DP, Hanson GS. Assessing the effects of school-based drug education: a six-year multi-level analysis of Project D.A.R.E. J. Res. Crime Delin. 1998;35:381-412.
[7] Shek DTL, Ma HK. Evaluation of the Project P.A.T.H.S. in Hong Kong: are the findings replicableacross different populations?Scientific WorldJournal 2010;10:178-81.
[8] Shek DTL, Sun RCF. Effectiveness of the Tier 1 Program of Project P.A.T.H.S.: findings based on three years of program implementation. Scientific World Journal 2010;10:1509-19.
[9] Shek DTL, Merrick, J. Training of potential program implementers of the Project P.A.T.H.S. in Hong Kong. Int. J. Adolesc. Med. Health 2010;22:341-3.

In: Drug Abuse in Hong Kong
Editors: D Shek, R Sun and J Merrick
ISBN: 978-1-61324-491-3
©2012 Nova Science Publishers, Inc.

Chapter 2

ENTHUSIASM-BASED OR EVIDENCE-BASED CHARITIES: PERSONAL REFLECTIONS

Daniel TL Shek[1,a,b,c,d,e]

[a]Department of Applied Social Sciences,
The Hong Kong Polytechnic University, Hong Kong, PRC
[b]Public Policy Research Institute,
The Hong Kong Polytechnic University, Hong Kong, PRC
[c]East China Normal University, Shanghai, PRC
[d]Kiang Wu Nursing College of Macau, Macau, PRC
[e]Division of Adolescent Medicine, Department of Pediatrics,
Kentucky Children's Hospital, University of Kentucky,
College of Medicine, Lexington, Kentucky, US

ABSTRACT

In different charitable foundations throughout the world, different approaches are used to allocate funding. As many projects with good will (i.e., enthusiasm-based charity) fail to help those who really need help, it is argued that evidence-based approach (i.e., charity guided by scientific evidence) represents the best strategy to support projects that can really help

---

[1]Correspondence: Professor Daniel TL Shek, PhD, FHKPS, BBS, JP, Chair Professor, Department of Applied Social Sciences, The Hong Kong Polytechnic University, Hunghom, Hong Kong. E-mail: daniel.shek@polyu.edu.hk.

the needy. Using this approach, scientific research findings are systematically used to: a) understand the nature of the problem and/or social needs; b) design appropriate intervention programs based on the best available evidence; and c) systematically evaluate the outcomes of the developed program. Using the Project P.A.T.H.S. funded by the Hong Kong Jockey Club Charities Trust as an example, the characteristics underlying this approach are outlined. The systematic use of scientific evidence in the Project P.A.T.H.S. is exemplary in different Chinese societies. This project provides much insight for charitable foundations and funding bodies locally and globally.

INTRODUCTION

In different parts of the world, charitable foundations have been set up by businessmen, corporations, and the public to help people in need. Most of the time, such foundations are seen as a sign of corporate social responsibility and an act of the company to serve the society. Some charitable organizations outside Hong Kong include the Bill and Melinda Gates Foundation (1), Ford Foundation (2), and Rockefeller Foundation (3). Similarly, there are many charitable foundations established in the private sector to meet the social needs of Hong Kong. Some examples include the Li Ka Sing Foundation, Hong Kong Bank Foundation, and Sun Hung Kai Properties-Kwok's Foundation. There are also foundations established by the Government to support welfare, education, and community projects, such as the Beat Drugs Fund and the Quality Education Fund.

Another important charitable organization in Hong Kong is the Hong Kong Jockey Club Charities Trust of the Hong Kong Jockey Club (4). As one of the largest racing organizations in the world, the Hong Kong Jockey Club is the sole authorized operator of horse race and football betting in Hong Kong. On behalf of the Hong Kong Lotteries Board, it also manages the Mark Six lotteries. One unique feature of the Hong Kong Jockey Club is that it upholds the not-for-profit gambling policy with the donation of surplus to charity and community projects (5). In the past decade, The Trust donated at an average of more than HK$1 billion each year. In 2006/07, a total of HK$1.05 billion was donated by the Trust to support 107 charities and community projects. These include community services projects (e.g., "CADENZA" which is a project serving old people and Project "P.A.T.H.S. to Adulthood" which is a project serving young people), education and training projects (e.g., The Hong Kong Jockey Club Education Fund and "READ and Write: A Jockey Club Learning Support Network" which is a project serving people with specific learning difficulties), medical and health projects (e.g., establishment of the Centre for Health Protection), and sport, recreational and cultural projects (e.g., establishment of the Jockey Club Kau Sai Chau Public Golf Course and a joint Sports Medicine and Health Sciences Centre with the involvement of The Chinese University of Hong Kong and The Hong Kong Polytechnic University).

FUND ALLOCATION POLICIES IN CHARITABLE FOUNDATIONS

It is both academically and practically important to know how funds are allocated in different charitable foundations and funding bodies. Based on the author's involvement in different high-level advisory committees and grant allocation committees of the Government of the Hong Kong Special Administrative Region, PRC and experiences in applying funding for welfare agencies from different charitable foundations, there are roughly seven approaches (some of which are not mutually exclusive) adopted by different charitable foundations and funding bodies in vetting applications and allocating funding:

- *Ease-based allocation approach:* Under this approach, funds are allocated based on convenience. Generally speaking, the grants available for allocation in a particular year will be allocated to as many applications as possible. One advantage of this approach is that it can guarantee that all applicants are happy because everybody gets something and the available money for allocation will be used up. One obvious disadvantage of this approach is that some applications with low quality may still get funding.
- *Eccentric and erratic allocation approach:* Under this approach, funds allocated are not based on consistent and rational principles. Most of the time, funding allocation depends on the taste and preference of the board members as well as the chairman of the board. As a result, funding allocation is often a product of politics and dynamics within the board rather than rational decision making.
- *Echo-based or envy-based allocation approach:* Utilizing this approach, funding allocation is based on a "follow-suit" manner. For example, if poverty is the main focus of the society recently and other charitable foundations fund projects on helping poor people, the foundation will

fund similar projects. In addition, as there is overt and/or covert competition among different charitable foundations, a foundation may envy of what other foundations are doing, hence funding projects of similar nature for unhealthy competition purpose.

- *Exposure-based allocation approach:* As some business corporations may regard publicity as the sole purpose of setting up charitable foundations, they may simply fund those projects that can bring public attention and promote exposure of the company. Under this approach, whether a project can serve as a good vehicle for publicity is the prime consideration in funding allocation.
- *Enthusiasm-based or emotion-based allocation approach:* For some social problems such as poverty and mental retardation, the miserable conditions of the clients will trigger the passion and emotions of the board members of charitable foundations. As such, the vetting committee may fund programs that are claimed to be able to improve the miserable conditions of the needy. In fact, programs may simply be funded out of enthusiasm and passion. Of course, developing programs to meet the needs of those living in miserable conditions isimportant. However, over-attention paid to the miserable conditions of the needy people at the expense of the real ability of the proposed program to improve the conditions of the needy may not be helpful to the needy at the end of the day. Obviously, we may have passion and good will but the proposed program may be a futile program. As pointed out by Bill and Melinda Gates Foundation, "philanthropy plays an important but limited role" but "science and technology have great potential to improve lives around the world" (1).
- *Error-based allocation approach:* Utilizing this approach, the funding body is funding programs that have been proved to be ineffective or programs that are not supported by evaluation findings. To avoid using this approach, adequate understanding of the literature on intervention research in human services is indispensable. Some examples will be given below to illustrate this approach.
- *Evidence-based allocation approach:* To help the needy in an effective manner, we need to understand the nature of their problems and needs, develop an intervention program which is based on best available evidence, and systematically evaluate the effectiveness of the implemented program. Obviously, science and scientific evidence play an important role in guiding charitable foundations in making important decisions. This approach is used in some of the major foundations. For

example, the Rockefeller Foundation explicitly states that "the Foundation vigorously and regularly measures impact and outcomes. Our initiatives specify clear time frames, identify anticipated results, and require monitoring and evaluation. This does not mean that we expect to solve the world's thorniest problems overnight. It does mean that Foundation-supported work defines hypotheses, articulates both short- and longer-term objectives, foresees and adapts to changing circumstances, and fully integrates verifiable methods of assessing progress"(3).

ENTHUSIASM-BASED AND ERROR-BASED ALLOCATION VERSUS EVIDENCE-BASED FUNDING POLICIES

In the literature on program evaluation, there are numerous examples showing that programs based on good will and passion may not be effective programs. Two examples are given here to illustrate the problems of enthusiasm-based and error-based allocation approaches. The first example is the Project D.A.R.E. (Drug Abuse Resistance Education) Program which was founded in 1983 in Los Angeles. This program was implemented in 75% of the school districts in the U.S.A. and in more than 43 countries around the world to help young people to resist pressure and to live drug and violence free lives. Unfortunately, several longitudinal studies have repeatedly showed that the program did not work (6,7). As pointed out by Rosenbaum and Hanson (8), "…can this popular school-based program prevent drug use at the stages in adolescent development when drugs become available and are widely used, namely, during the high school years? Unfortunately, the answer to the question is 'no' " (p. 404). Obviously, popularity and enthusiasm alone do not guarantee program success.

The second example is programs involving visits to prisons so as to deter young people from committing crimes. In such programs (e.g., Scare Straight), it is typically assumed that organization of visits to prison facilities for juvenile delinquents and children at risk of delinquency would deter the likelihood of offence, hence lowering the crime rates for the young people concerned (9). Unfortunately, the review conducted by Petrosino, Petrosino-Turpin, and Buehler (10) showed that such programs could not deter young people from committing crimes. In fact, the reviewers concluded that "programmes like 'Sacred Straight' are likely to have a harmful effect and increase delinquency relative to doing nothing at all to the same youths. Given these results, agencies that permit such programmes must rigorously evaluate them not only to ensure that they are doing what they purport to do (prevent crime) – but at the very least they do not cause more harm than good" (p. 2).

Rubin and Babbie (11) pointed out that there are many ways of generating knowledge claims. First, we develop knowledge claims via tenacity such as cultural beliefs. One example is the cultural belief that "a dutiful son is a product of the rod" which endorses the importance of harsh punishment in child rearing. The second way is common sense such as ventilating emotion is important for an emotionally distressed person. The third way is deriving knowledge claims based on authority such as university professors and government officials. For example, under the influence of Newton, people believe that there are physical laws that are universal in any contexts (but these universal laws become shaky under Einstein's theory). The fourth way is to develop knowledge claims through a priori method or logic. Based on certain premise (e.g., poverty leads to juvenile delinquency), one can logically deduce certain knowledge claims (e.g., juvenile delinquency is higher in poor relative to non-poor adolescents). Finally, knowledge claims can be derived from the scientific method. Through induction and deduction, one can verify the validity of the deduced hypotheses. Among these methods of developing knowledge claims, the scientific method is the preferred approach of generating knowledge claims.

According to Gambrill (12), there are two ways of understanding the world and generating knowledge claims. The first way is authority-based practice that generates authority-based knowledge. Under this approach, there is reliance on authority (such as experts and authority in the field) as the ultimate standard and false knowledge where belief that is not true and not questioned is generated. In addition, authority-based practice is in fact pseudoscience with several characteristics, including discouragement of critical scrutiny of knowledge claims, use rituals of science without substance, reliance on anecdotal experience, lack of skepticism, treat open mind as uncritical mind, ignoring negative evidence, and upholding beliefs which are not verifiable.

On the other hand, evidence-based practice emphasizes the importance of utilizing evidence in providing service which usually involves five steps (13). In Step 1, issues related to intervention are formulated in terms of answerable questions. In Step 2, the practitioner searches the literature to locate the best evidence on the problem under focus. In Step 3, the worker critically appraises the evidence in terms of its validity, reliability, and clinical applicability. In Step 4, the best evidence that has been critically scrutinized would be implemented. In Step 5, clinical performance would be evaluated. Gambrill (14) further pointed out the there are several core values underlying the intellectual base of evidence-based practice. These include courage (evaluate knowledge claims in a bold manner), curiosity (deep interest in knowledge), intellectual empathy (accurately presenting the views of others), humility (acknowledging one's limitations), integrity (no double standards), and persistence (endurance in view of adversity). Gambrill (12) clearly stated that "different ways of knowing differ in the extent to which they highlight uncertainty and are designed to weed out biases and distortions that may influence assumptions" (p. 343). Obviously, systematic use of research findings in understanding the problem encountered (e.g., adolescent substance abuse), developing appropriate intervention program, and collecting evaluation data in a systematic manner to assess the implementation of the program and outcomes are important.

PROJECT P.A.T.H.S. AND EVIDENCE-BASED POSITIVE YOUTH DEVELOPMENT PROGRAM

A survey of the literature shows that there are worrying trends and phenomena related to the development of adolescents in Hong Kong, such as mental health problems, abuse of psychotropic substances, adolescent suicide, school violence, and drop in family solidarity(15). As such, primary prevention programs targeting specific adolescent developmental problems and positive youth development programs are called for. However, research findings show that there are very few systematic and multi-year positive youth development programs in Hong Kong. Even if such programs exist, they commonly deal with isolated problems and issues in adolescent development (i.e., deficits-oriented programs) and they are relatively short-term in nature. In addition, systematic and long-term evaluation of the available programs does not exist.

To promote holistic development among adolescents in Hong Kong, the Hong Kong Jockey Club Charities Trust has approved a total of HK$750 million to launch a project entitled "P.A.T.H.S. to Adulthood: A Jockey Club Youth Enhancement Scheme". The word "P.A.T.H.S." denotes Positive Adolescent Training through Holistic Social Programmes. The Trust has invited academics of five universities in Hong Kong to form a Research Team with The Hong Kong Polytechnic University as the lead institution and the author as the Principal Investigator to develop a multi-year universal positive youth development program to promote holistic adolescent development in Hong Kong.

To achieve these objectives, a curriculum-based program (Tier 1 Program) was developed. The design of the program and constructs included in the program were based on a thorough and systematic review of the scientific literature (16). In particular, focus was put on the work of Catalano, Berglund, Ryan, Lonczak, and Hawkins (17) who found that only 25 programs out of 75 positive youth development programs under review were successful and 15 positive youth development constructs were identified in the successful programs. These constructs are presented as follows:

1. Promotion of Bonding: Development of the program participants' relationship with healthy adults and positive peers in the extra-familial contexts (school, community and cultural contexts) and caregivers and significant-others in the intra-familial context.
2. Cultivation of Resilience: Promotion of capacity for adapting to change and stressful events in healthy and adaptive ways.
3. Promotion of Social Competence: Training the program participants' interpersonal skills (including communication, assertiveness, refusal and resistance, conflict resolution, and interpersonal negotiation) and providing opportunities to practice such skills.
4. Promotion of Emotional Competence: Training the program participants' skills to recognize feelings in oneself and others (including empathy), skills to express feelings, skills to manage emotional reactions or impulses (delay of gratification and frustration tolerance), and emotional self-management strategies.
5. Promotion of Cognitive Competence: Developing the program participants' cognitive abilities, processes or outcomes, including academic performance, logical thinking, critical thinking, problem-solving, decision making, planning and goal setting, and self-talk.
6. Promotion of Behavioral Competence: Cultivation of verbal communication (making requests and positive response to criticisms), non-verbal communication and taking action skills, and providing reinforcement for the effective behavior choices and action pattern.
7. Promotion of Moral Competence: Development of a sense of right and wrong and respect for rules and standards as well as social justice.
8. Cultivation of Self-Determination: Promoting the program participants' sense of autonomy, independent thinking, or self-advocacy.
9. Promotion of Spirituality: Helps the program participants to develop purpose and meaning in life, hope, or beliefs in a higher power.
10. Development of Self-Efficacy: Promoting the program participants' coping and mastery skills and changing their negative self-efficacy expectancies or self-defeating cognitions.

11. Development of a Clear and Positive Identity: Promotion of healthy identity formation and achievement, including positive identification with one's social or ethnic identity.
12. Promotion of Beliefs in the Future: Helping program participants to develop future potential goals, choices or options.
13. Provision of Recognition for Positive Behavior: Developing systems for rewarding, recognizing or reinforcing participants' positive behavior such as prosocial behavior or positive changes in behavior.
14. Providing Opportunities for Prosocial Involvement: Designing activities and events for program participants to make positive contribution to groups.
15. Fostering Prosocial Norms: Encouraging program participants to develop clear and explicit standards for prosocial engagement.

Furthermore, based on the literature review, several assertions are maintained in the conceptual model underlying the proposed program in the present project(16).As far as curriculum development is concerned, the following principles are maintained in the process of designing the Tier 1 Program after a thorough review of the literature (18):

- Principle 1: The program is a comprehensive universal program that utilizes a wide range of positive youth development constructs that have been identified in the effective programs.
- Principle 2: Relevant theoretical models and research findings in both Western and Chinese contexts are used to guide the development of the program.
- Principle 3: Holistic adolescent development in different domains (physical, psychological, social, and spiritual domains) is focused upon.
- Principle 4: Both adolescent developmental assets and developmental problems (e.g., drug, sex, delinquent, violence, lifestyle, money spending and mental health issues) are considered in the process.
- Principle 5: The proposed program content is developmentally appropriate.
- Principle 6: Relevant cultural elements are included in the program.
- Principle 7: Multi-year intervention programs rather than one-shot programs are designed.
- Principle 8: Proper and adequate training is planned for the teachers and social workers who implement the programs.

- Principle 9: Relevant teaching strategies and methods (e.g., using peers to demonstrate skills and change norms) are used to maximize the learning effects.
- Principle 10: Active participation and involvement of the students are emphasized.
- Principle 11: Besides classroom activities, programs outside the classroom are developed.
- Principle 12: Generalization of the competence developed to the real-life world is emphasized.
- Principle 13: Students are involved in the design of the program activities.
- Principle 14: Relevant issues (e.g., gender differences, school differences, and class differences) are considered in the program design.
- Principle 15: Besides changing the students, attempts to change the families (e.g., encouraging parental involvement) and schools (e.g., school improvement and reorganization initiatives included) are included.
- Principle 16: Ongoing evaluation at all stages is carried out.

As training of potential program implementers is an important part of the project, training programs were also designed based on a thorough review of the literature. Based on a critical review of the studies in this area, several principles governing training of the potential program implementers are maintained in the study (19):

- Principle 1: Design of the training program is based on training theories/models.
- Principle 2: Acquisition of knowledge about adolescents and the program in the training program.
- Principle 3: Acquisition of knowledge about the curriculum structure of the program in the training program.
- Principle 4: Cultivation of appropriate implementation skills in the training program.
- Principle 5: Cultivation of self-reflection skills in the training program.
- Principle 6: Encouragement of workers to be role models.
- Principle 7: Promotion of motivation of the trainees.
- Principle 8: Promotion of self-efficacy of the trainees.
- Principle 9: Provision of opportunities for demonstration and practice.
- Principle 10: Provision of adequate training time.

- Principle 11: Consideration of cultural context in the design of the training program.
- Principle 12: Evaluation of the training program.

Finally, based on literature review, an evaluation design based on multiple evaluation strategies and the principle of triangulation is adopted with the following evaluation methods (20):

1. Objective Outcome Evaluation: Evaluation findings based on a one-group pretest-posttest design (21) and a randomized group trial were collected.
2. Subjective Outcome Evaluation: Both students and program implementers were invited to complete subjective outcome evaluation forms after completion of the program (22,23). Convergence between subjective outcome evaluation and objective outcome evaluation findings was also examined (24).
3. Process Evaluation: Systematic observations were carried out in randomly selected schools to understand the program implementation details (25).
4. Interim Evaluation: To understand the process of implementation, interim evaluation was conducted by randomly selecting half of the participating schools (26).
5. Qualitative Evaluation (Focus Groups Based on Students): Focus groups involving students based on schools randomly selected from the participating schools were carried out.
6. Qualitative Evaluation (Focus Groups Based on Program Implementers): Focus groups involving instructors based on schools randomly selected from the participating schools were carried out.
7. Qualitative Evaluation (In-depth Interviews with Program Implementers): Prolonged in-depth interviews with two teachers were carried out.
8. Qualitative Evaluation (Case Study Based on Focus Groups): A case study based on 7 schools participating in the Secondary 1 Program of the Full Implementation Phase was conducted.
9. Qualitative Evaluation (Student Logs): Four students were invited to reflect on their experiences after joining the classes and application of things learned to real life.
10. Qualitative Evaluation (Student Products): Students' weekly diaries were collected after completion of the program (27).

An integration of research findings collected from different sources shows that there is support for the effectiveness of the Project P.A.T.H.S.. The details of the evaluation findings supporting the Project P.A.T.H.S. can be seen in the website of the project (http://www.paths.hk).

TOWARDS EVIDENCE-BASED WELFARE AND HUMAN SERVICE IN HONG KONG

Shek, Lam, and Tsoi (28) showed that evidence-based social work practice was very primitive in Hong Kong and there were many obstacles involved. Of course, one good way to promote evidence-based practice is that charitable foundations adopt an evidence-based approach in vetting and funding research proposals and attempts that systematically utilize research findings in understanding the problem area, developing evidence-based programs and evaluating the effectiveness of the developed programs are duly recognized. As members of the funding allocation committees in charitable foundations and other funding bodies, one should realize that there are six possible types of community and welfare programs with different levels of effectiveness: a) ineffective or harmful intervention; b) intervention unlikely to be beneficial; c) intervention with unknown effectiveness; d) intervention with both benefits and adverse effects; e) intervention likely to be beneficial; and f) intervention is effective which is reflected by clear evidence form controlled trials. For funding bodies and charitable foundations, it is important to routinely fund projects that are promising and systematically utilizing research findings to understand the nature of the issue to be tackled, develop the intervention programs and to systematically evaluate the programs. Obviously, the Project P.A.T.H.S. can be regarded as an exemplary program that can instill paradigm shifts in charitable foundations and funding bodies locally and globally.

ACKNOWLEDGMENTS

The preparation for this paper and the Project P.A.T.H.S. were financially supported by The Hong Kong Jockey Club Charities Trust.

REFERENCES

[1] Bill and Melinda Gates Foundation. Accessed 2011 Feb 11. Available at: http://www.gatesfoundation.org/Pages/home.aspx.
[2] Ford Foundation. Accessed 2011 Feb 11. Available at: http://www.fordfound.org.
[3] Rockefeller Foundation.Accessed 2011 Feb 11. Available at: http://www.rockfound.org.
[4] Hong Kong Jockey Club Charities Trust. Accessed 2011 Feb 11. Available at: http://charities.hkjc.com/charities/charities-overview/ english/charities-trust.aspx.
[5] The Hong Kong Jockey Club. Responsible gambling policy and practices. Accessed 2011 Feb 11. Available at: http://corporate.hkjc.com/corporate/rgp/english/index.aspx.
[6] Ennett ST, Tobler NS, Ringwalt CL, Flewelling RL. How effective is drug resistance education? A meta-analysis of Project DARE outcome evaluations. Am. J.Pub. Health1994;84:1394-401.
[7] West SL, O'Neil KK. Project DARE outcome effectiveness revisited. Am. J. Pub. Health2004;94:1027-9.
[8] Rosenbaum DP, Hanson GS. Assessing the effects of school-based drug education: a six-year multi-level analysis of Project D.A.R.E. J. Res. Crime Delin.1998;35:381-412.
[9] Petrosino A, Petrosino-Turpin C, Finkenauer JO.Well-meaning programs can have harmful effects! Lessons from experiments in Scared Straight and other like programs. Crime Delin. 2000;46:354-79.
[10] Petrosino A, Petrosino-Turpin C, Buehler J. Scared Straight and other juvenile awareness programs for preventing juvenile delinquency: a systematic review of the randomized experimental evidence. Ann. Am. Acad. Pol. Soc. Sci.2003;589(1):41-62.
[11] Rubin A, Babbie, E. Research methods for social work. Delmont, CA: Thomson Learning, 2008.
[12] Gambrill E. Evidence-based practice: an alternative to authority-based practice. Fam. Soc.1999;80:341-50.
[13] SackettDL, RichardsonWS, Rosenberg W, Haynes RB. Evidence-based medicine: How to practice and teach EBM. New York: Churchill Livingstone, 1997.
[14] Gambrill E. Evidence-based practice and policy: choice ahead. Res. Soc. Work Pract. 2006;16:338-57.
[15] Shek DTL. Adolescent developmental issues in Hong Kong: relevance to positive youth development programs in Hong Kong. Int. J. Adolesc. Med. Health 2006;18:341-54.
[16] Shek DTL. Conceptual framework underlying the development of a positive youth development program in Hong Kong. Int. J. Adolesc. Med. Health 2006;18:303-14.
[17] Catalano RF, Berglund ML, Ryan JAM, Lonczak HS, Hawkins JD. Positive youth development in the United States: research findings on evaluations of positive youth development programs. Prev Treatment 2002. Accessed 2011 Feb 11. Available at: http://www.aspe.hhs.gov/hsp/positiveyouthdev99/.
[18] Shek DTL, Ma HK. Design of a positive youth development program in Hong Kong. Int. J. Adolesc. Med. Health 2006;18:315-27.
[19] Shek DTL, Wai CLY. Training workers implementing adolescent prevention and positive youth development programs: what have we learned from the literature? Adolesc. 2008;43(172):823-45.

[20] Shek DTL, Siu AMH. Evaluation of a positive youth development program in Hong Kong: issues, principles and design. Int. J. Adolesc. Med. Health 2006;18:329-39.
[21] Shek DTL. Effectiveness of the Tier 1 Program of the Project P.A.T.H.S.: preliminary objective and subjective outcome evaluation findings. ScientificWorld Journal 2006;6:1466-74.
[22] Shek DTL, Ma HK. Subjective outcome evaluation of the Project P.A.T.H.S.: findings based on the program participants. ScientificWorld Journal 2007;7:47-55.
[23] Shek DTL, Siu AMH, Lee TY. Subjective outcome evaluation of the Project P.A.T.H.S.: findings based on the perspective of the program implementers.ScientificWorld Journal 2007;7:195-203.
[24] Shek DTL, Lee TY, Siu AMH, Ma HK. Convergence of subjective outcome and objective outcome evaluation findings: insights based on the Project P.A.T.H.S.ScientificWorld Journal2007;7:258-67.
[25] Shek DTL, Ma HK, Lui JHY, Lung DWM. Process evaluation of the Tier 1 Program of the Project P.A.T.H.S.ScientificWorld Journal2006;6:2264-73.
[26] Shek DTL, SunRCF. Implementation of the Tier 1 Program of the Project P.A.T.H.S.: interim evaluation findings. ScientificWorld Journal 2006;6:2274-84.
[27] Shek DTL, Lee TY, Siu A, Lam CM. Qualitative evaluation of the Project P.A.T.H.S. based on the perceptions of the program participants. ScientificWorld Journal 2006;6:2254-63.
[28] Shek DTL, Lam MC, TsoiKW. Evidence-based practice in Hong Kong. In: Thyer B, Kazi MAF,eds. International perspectives on evidence-based practice in social work. London: Venture Press, 2004:167-81.

In: Drug Abuse in Hong Kong
Editors: D Shek, R Sun and J Merrick

ISBN: 978-1-61324-491-3
©2012 Nova Science Publishers, Inc.

Chapter 3

SCHOOL DRUG TESTING: A CRITICAL REVIEW OF THE LITERATURE

Daniel TL Shek[1,a,b,c,d,e]

[a]Department of Applied Social Sciences,
The Hong Kong Polytechnic University, Hong Kong, PRC
[b]Public Policy Research Institute,
The Hong Kong Polytechnic University, Hong Kong, PRC
[c]East China Normal University, Shanghai, PRC
[d]Kiang Wu Nursing College of Macau, Macau, PRC
[e]Division of Adolescent Medicine, Department of Pediatrics,
Kentucky Children's Hospital, University of Kentucky,
College of Medicine, Lexington, Kentucky, US

ABSTRACT

This chapter explores the question of whether school drug testing is an effective solution to tackle adolescent substance abuse problem. Research studies in major academic databases and the Internet websites are reviewed. Several observations are highlighted from the review: a) there are few research studies in this area, particularly in different Chinese contexts; b) the

---

[1]Correspondence: Professor Daniel TL Shek, PhD, FHKPS, BBS, JP, Chair Professor, Department of Applied Social Sciences, The Hong Kong Polytechnic University, Hunghom, Hong Kong. E-mail: daniel.shek@polyu.edu.hk.

quality of the existing studies was generally low; and c) research findings supporting the effectiveness of school drug testing were mixed. Methodological issues underlying quantitative and qualitative evaluation studies of the effectiveness of school drug testing are discussed.

INTRODUCTION

A survey of the websites of several international organizations (e.g., Office on Drugs and Crime of the United Nations, International Narcotics Control Board, National Institute of Drug Abuse in the United States, and European Monitoring Center for Drugs and Drug Addiction) shows that illicit drug use is a thorny global problem to be resolved. Probably because of the influence of popular culture and youth sub-culture, substance abuse among young people has also become an acute global problem(1,2). With reference to the findings reported in some of the major databases on adolescent development such as Monitoring the Future, Youth Risk Behavior Surveillance(YRBS) and National Household Survey on Drug Abuse (NHSDA), adolescent substance abuse is a concern for policy makers and health professionals(3). From the results of the 2008 National Survey on Drug Use and Health, it was found that 9.3 percent of youths aged 12 to 17 were current illicit drug users(4).

To tackle the gradual worsening of adolescent drug abuse, school drug testing has been adopted in some Western countries to cope with the problem. In 1995, the US Supreme Court approved drug testing for student athletes in public high schools. In 2002, the US Supreme Court broadened the ruling to include all students taking part in competitions against students at other schools in after-school activities(5). Ever since its inception, there has been much debate on the necessity and value of student drug testing, particularly its effectiveness. Roche et al. (6) reviewed the theories, assumptions, and limitations of the underlying rationales for school drug testing. They also reviewed some of the studies in the field and concluded that quality of the studies was generally low. Although the study of Roche et al. (6) is a pioneering attempt to review some of the studies in the field, there are three limitations. First, the studies under review were not exhaustive. Some of the studies reported in academic journals and the Internet were not included. Second, although the quality of the studies under review was mentioned in the paper, the details (e.g., problems of the design, methodology and data analyses, biased conclusions …etc) were not included. Third, the findings supporting and not supporting the effectiveness of school drug testing were not separately reported. Against this background, the present study attempted to review the literature in which the findings supporting and not supporting the effectiveness of school drug testing were separated. Besides, quality of the studies was evaluated in details. Finally, methodological issues intrinsic to quantitative and qualitative studies of the effectiveness of school drug testing were discussed.

SEARCH

A systematic review of the major academic databases (including PsycINFO, Social Work Abstracts, Medline, CINAHL, and Sociological Abstracts) was carried out with the use of the following search terms: "random drug test", "drug testing", "school drug testing", and "drug detection". In addition, empirical studies reported in the websites in the Internet were also reviewed using the above terms. Some of the authoritative websites on school drug testing are presented in Table 1. The studies under review in this study are outlined in Appendix 1.

Table 1. Internet websites on school drug testing

Resource	Website
American Civil Liberties Union - A Test You Can't Study For	http://www.aclu.org/drugpolicy/testing/10845res20021021.html
Drug Policy Alliance Network	http://www.drugpolicy.org/law/drugtesting/students/
Monitoring the Future survey	http://www.monitoringthefuture.org
Office of Safe and Drug-free Schools, U.S. Department of Education	http://www.ed.gov/about/offices/list/osdfs/index.html
Prevention Resources and Information on Drug Education (PRIDE)	http://www.prideprevention.org/
Student Drug Testing Coalition	http://www.studentdrugtesting.org/
Students for Sensible Drug Policy (SSDP)	http://www.DAREgeneration.com
The Association for Addiction Professionals	http://www.naadac.org/

Table 2. Studies supporting school drug testing

Study	Study Design	Setting	Sample	Intervention	Outcomes assessed	Findings
Combs and Ryan (1990)	Cross-sectional survey and in-depth interview	21 Intercollegiate teams, UCLA, USA	500 student athletes with drug testing 124 untested student athletes	Mandatory drug testing program	Identification of students' drug use Students' reported continued drug use	Drug testing effective: - identification of drug users - prevention of continued drug use Reduced drug use found in most of drug-using athletes
Coombs and Coombs (1991)	Cross-sectional survey and in-depth interview	21 Intercollegiate teams, UCLA, USA	500 student athletes	Mandatory drug testing program	Students' morale and psychological well-being	Most students reported not affected by drug testing Positive benefits: - promote awareness of negative drug effects - offer socially acceptable way to resist drug use - enhance athletic and academic performance
DuPont, Campbell, and Mazza (2002)	Cross-sectional survey	9 high schools, USA	School administrators, Counselors, Athletic directors, Drug prevention coordinators	Student drug testing	Students' reported drug use Disciplinary problems	Decreased students' illicit drug use Reduced disciplinary problems: - lowered detention rate for disruptive behavior - reduced student arrests

Study	Study Design	Setting	Sample	Intervention	Outcomes assessed	Findings
McKinney (2002)	Cross-sectional survey	83 high schools, Indiana, USA	83 high school principals	Mandatory, random drug testing in 1999-2000	Drug testing suspended 2000-2001: Students' reported illicit drug use; Students' alcohol use; Students' suspension or expulsion due to drug or alcohol use	Increased illicit drug use; Increased alcohol use; Statistically significant increase in students' suspension or expulsion
McKinney (2003)	Cross-sectional survey McKinney's (2002) follow-up	59 high schools, Indiana, USA	59 high school principals	Mandatory, random, suspicion-less drug testing program	Students' reported drug and alcohol use when drug testing re-implemented	Drug testing discouraged students' drug and alcohol use; Decreased students' drug and alcohol use
McKinney (2005)	Cross-sectional survey McKinney's (2003) follow-up	56 high schools, Indiana, USA	56 high school principals	Mandatory, random, suspicion-less drug testing program	Students' reported illicit drug use; Students' participation in athletic program; Students' academic performance	Reduced students' drug use; Rise in student participation in athletic program; Schools with drug testing: - above average in state graduation test - graduation rate higher than state average

Table 2. (Continued)

Study	Study Design	Setting	Sample	Intervention	Outcomes assessed	Findings
McKinney (2005)	Cross-sectional survey McKinney's (2003) follow-up	56 high schools, Indiana, USA	56 high school principals	Mandatory, random, suspicion-less drug testing program	Students' reported illicit drug use Students' participation in athletic program Students' academic performance	Reduced students' drug use Rise in student participation in athletic program Schools with drug testing: - above average in state graduation test - graduation rate higher than state average
Mason (2003)	Cross-sectional survey	High schools, USA	620 high school students	Drug testing program	Students' attitude toward drug testing	Neutral attitude on drug testing in most students More positive attitude found in younger students Drug testing less accepting in students with stronger pro-drug attitude
Goldberg, Elliot, MacKinnon, Moe, Kuehl, Nohre, and Lockwood (2003)	Longitudinal survey 1999-2000	2 high schools, Oregon, USA	Athletes vs. non-athletes: T1: 276 vs. 507 T2: 159 vs. 338	Mandatory drug testing program for student athletes	Students' past 30-day drug use Students' attitude and beliefs on drug testing	Reduced student athletes' past 30-day drug use Positive attitude toward drug testing in intervention and control groups

Study	Study Design	Setting	Sample	Intervention	Outcomes assessed	Findings
Evans, Reader, Liss, Wiens, and Roy (2006)	Cross-sectional survey conducted before drug testing implementation	2 rural high schools, North Florida, USA	1,011 students from 9th to 11th grade	Random suspicion-less drug testing program	Students' perceived fairness of drug testing policy. Students' predicted effectiveness to reduce drug use	Perceived drug problem found as robust predictor of perceived policy fairness. Most students perceived that drug testing would be effective to reduce drug use
Evans-Whipp, Bond, Toumbourou, and Catalano (2007)	Cross-sectional survey	International Youth Development Study data 2003: 104 schools, Washington, USA 101 schools, Victoria, Australia	Washington: 1,934 students 1,886 parents Victoria: 1,942 students 1,858 parents	Drug testing program	Students' reported drug use. Parents' and students' awareness of policy	Drug testing policy associated with decreased student drug use. The message of harm reduction associated with reduced drug use. Parents and students aware of school policy orientation
Goldberg, Elliot, MacKinnon, Moe, Kuehl, Yoon, Taylor, and Williams (2007)	Two-year prospective randomized controlled study of a single cohort	14 school districts, Oregon, USA	653 students in 5 high schools with drug testing. 743 students in 6 control schools	Random drug and alcohol testing in high school athletes	Students' past-year reported drug use. Students' past-month reported drug use	Reduced students' past-year drug use in 2 of 4 follow-ups

Table 2. (Continued)

Study	Study Design	Setting	Sample	Intervention	Outcomes assessed	Findings
Barrington(2008)	Quasi-experimental mixed-methods sequential explanatory design	2 rural, low-income public secondary school districts, USA	1,048 high school students from 6th to 12th grade, and four school administrators	Voluntary, randomized, student drug testing program	Drug testing efficacy	Qualitative findings: - students with intensive drug abuse service needs identified - enhance school bonding and connectedness
Ringwalt, Vincus, Ennett, Hanley, Bowling, Yacoubian, and Rohrbach(2009)	Cross-sectional survey in spring 2005	School districts from a national random sample, USA	1,612 drug prevention coordinators from 1,922 school districts	Suspicion-less random drug testing implemented in 205 school districts	School districts' responses to students' first positive drug test	Appropriate responses: - refer students and parents to meet with school personnel and counselor - require students to receive drug education and treatment

Table 3. Studies not supporting school drug testing

Study	Study Design	Setting	Sample	Intervention	Outcomes assessed	Findings
Combs and Ryan (1990)	Cross-sectional survey and in-depth interview	21 Intercollegiate teams, UCLA, USA	500 student athletes with drug testing 124 untested student athletes	Drug testing program	Identification of students' drug use Students' reported continued drug use	Elevated level of drug use reported in some students Ways to avoid detection of drugs reported in some students

Study	Study Design	Setting	Sample	Intervention	Outcomes assessed	Findings
Coombs and Coombs (1991)	Cross-sectional survey and in-depth interview	21 Intercollegiate teams, UCLA, USA	500 student athletes	Mandatory drug testing for intercollegiate athletes	Students' morale and psychological well-being Improvement in drug testing experience	Negative feelings reported: - embarrassed and humiliated Suggested improvements: - orientation and education - comfortable testing setting - reasonable objectives - rigorous testing standards
McKinney (2002)	Cross-sectional survey	83 high schools, Indiana, USA	83 high school principals	Mandatory, drug testing in 1999-2000	Students' reported illicit drug use in 2000-2001	Students' reported drug use unchanged
McKinney (2003)	Cross-sectional survey McKinney's (2002) follow-up	59 high schools, Indiana, USA	59 high school principals	Mandatory, random drug testing program	Students' reported drug use when drug testing re-implemented	Reported drug use unchanged in some students
Goldberg, Elliot, MacKinnon, Moe, Kuehl, Nohre, and Lockwood (2003)	Longitudinal survey 1999-2000	2 high schools, Oregon, USA	Athletes vs. non-athletes: T1: 276 vs. 507 T2: 159 vs. 338	Mandatory drug testing program for student athletes	New drug use Students' attitude and beliefs on drug testing Students' attitude toward school	No difference in new drug use between control and intervention schools Beliefs in reduced risk of drugs increased Negative attitude toward school increased

Table 3. (Continued)

Study	Study Design	Setting	Sample	Intervention	Outcomes assessed	Findings
Yamaguchi, Johnston, and O'Malley(2003).	Cross-sectional national survey from 1998 to 2001	Monitoring the Future study Youth, Education, and Society study USA	Monitoring the Future study: 76,000 students from 8th, 10th, and 12th grades	School drug testing program	Prevalence of students' reported illicit drug use Rate of students' reported marijuana use	Drug testing not associated with: - prevalence of students' reported illicit drug use - rate of drug use in experienced marijuana users
Evans, Reader, Liss, Wiens, and Roy (2006)	Cross-sectional survey conducted before drug testing implementation	2 rural high schools, North Florida, USA	1,011 students from 9th to 11th grade	Random suspicion-less drug testing program	Students' perceived fairness of drug testing policy	Better acceptance of drug testing should address: - students' perceptions of peer drug use - drug testing accuracy - equitability of drug testing consequences
Goldberg, Elliot, MacKinnon, Moe, Kuehl, Yoon, Taylor, and Williams (2007)	Two-year prospective randomized controlled study of a single cohort	14 school districts, Oregon, USA	653 students in 5 high schools with drug testing 743 students in 6 control schools	Random drug and alcohol testing in high school athletes	Students' past-month reported drug use	No deterrent effects for past-month drug use in any of the 4 follow-ups Increased risk factors for future drug use

Study	Study Design	Setting	Sample	Intervention	Outcomes assessed	Findings
Barrington(2008)	Quasi-experimental, mixed-methods sequential explanatory design	2 rural, low-income public secondary school districts, USA	1,048 high school students from 6th to 12th grade, and four school administrators	Voluntary, randomized, student drug testing program	Students' reported drug use	Quantitative finding: No significant impact on students' reported drug use
What Works Clearinghouse (2008, May)	Review of Goldberg et al.'s (2007) study	14 school districts, Oregon, USA	653 students in 5 schools with drug testing 743 students in 6 control schools	Random drug and alcohol testing in high school athletes	Sample attrition rate Demographic data of sample	Goldberg et al.'s (2007) study inconclusive findings: - high attrition rate - biased sampling
Ringwalt,Vincus,Ennett,Hanley,Bowling, Yacoubian, and Rohrbach(2009)	Cross-sectional survey in spring 2005	School districts from a national random sample, USA	1,612 drug prevention coordinators from 1,922 school districts	Random drug testing in 205 school districts	School districts' responses to students' first positive drug test	Less appropriate responses: - inform law enforcement, - suspension from athletic team or school

Table 4. Quality of studies under review

Study	Study Design	Comments on the Study
Combs and Ryan (1990)	Cross-sectional survey and in-depth interview	No cause-effect inference could be drawn from the findings Details of group comparison not clear Samples were not randomly drawn Psychometric properties of the assessment tools unclear Qualitative orientation of the study not clear Unclear about how ideological preoccupation and biases were dealt with Qualitative analysis procedures unclear Limitations of the study not properly addressed
Coombs and Coombs (1991)	Cross-sectional survey and in-depth interview	No cause-effect inference could be drawn from the findings Psychometric properties of the assessment tools unclear Samples were not randomly drawn Descriptive statistics were the main form of analyses Qualitative orientation of the study not clear Qualitative analysis procedures unclear Unclear about how ideological preoccupation and biases were dealt with Limitations of the study not properly addressed
DuPont, Campbell, and Mazza (2002)	Cross-sectional survey (quantitative and qualitative data collected)	No cause-effect inference could be drawn from the findings Psychometric properties of the assessment tools unclear Samples were not randomly drawn Descriptive statistics were the main form of analyses Qualitative orientation of the study not clear Unclear about how ideological preoccupation and biases were dealt with Qualitative data analysis procedures not clear Limitations of the study not properly addressed

Study	Study Design	Comments on the Study
McKinney (2002)	Cross-sectional survey	No cause-effect inference could be drawn from the findings Psychometric properties of the assessment tools unclear Samples were not randomly drawn Descriptive statistics were the main form of analyses Research report is very brief Findings on the impact of random student drug-testing programs are not robust – many confounding factors would affect the results Limitations of the study not properly addressed
McKinney (2003)	Cross-sectional survey McKinney's (2002) follow-up	No cause-effect inference could be drawn from the findings Psychometric properties of the assessment tools unclear Samples were not randomly drawn Procedures for data collection not clear Descriptive statistics were the main form of analyses Research report is very brief Effect of re-implementation of drug-testing programs not properly evaluated Alternative explanations not properly evaluated Limitations of the study not properly addressed
McKinney (2005)	Cross-sectional survey McKinney's (2003) follow-up	No cause-effect inference could be drawn from the findings Psychometric properties of the assessment tools unclear Samples were not randomly drawn Hypotheses of the study are not clearly stated The procedures are not systematically presented Descriptive statistics were the main form of analyses No details about inferential statistics used Research report is very brief Alternative explanations of the findings were not discussed Limitations of the study not properly addressed The conclusion that drug testing policies are effective is not adequately supported by the evidence presented

Table 4. (Continued)

Study	Study Design	Comments on the Study
Mason (2003)	Cross-sectional survey	No cause-effect inference could be drawn from the findings Psychometric properties of the assessment tools unclear Samples were not randomly drawn Sample errors associated with the percentage data not properly addressed
Goldberg, Elliot, MacKinnon, Moe, Kuehl, Nohre, and Lockwood (2003)	Longitudinal survey 1999-2000	Longitudinal design commendable Inclusion of a comparison school is methodologically superior No cause-effect inference could be drawn from the findings Some of the measures had low internal consistency Validity of the outcome measures in both groups not clear Samples were not randomly drawn Only one experimental school and one control school was involved Only mandatory drug testing among the athletes was focused upon Only quantitative data were collected Subject attrition effect not fully explored
Evans, Reader, Liss, Wiens, and Roy (2006)	Cross-sectional survey conducted before drug testing implementation	No cause-effect inference could be drawn from the findings Reliability of the 10-item measure was not particularly high Validity of the 10-item measure is not clear Samples were not randomly drawn Predictors of fairness attitude and policy effectiveness belief were examined Limitations of the study discussed Only quantitative data were collected
Evans-Whipp, Bond, Toumbourou, and Catalano (2007)	Cross-sectional survey	No cause-effect inference could be drawn from the findings Students, parents and administrators were recruited Large sample size in different samples Random and representative samples drawn Psychometric properties of the instruments not clear Both descriptive and inferential statistical analyses were conducted, Limitations of the study discussed, Only quantitative data were collected

Study	Study Design	Comments on the Study
Goldberg, Elliot, MacKinnon, Moe, Kuehl, Yoon, Taylor, and Williams (2007)	Two-year prospective randomized controlled study of a single cohort	Two-year prospective randomized controlled study Reliability of measures acceptable Validity of measures not clear Limitations of the study discussed Linear mixed models not employed Only quantitative data were collected
Barrington(2008)	Quasi-experimental mixed-methods sequential explanatory design	A mixed-method design was adopted Validated measures were used Samples were not randomly drawn Qualitative orientation of the study not clear Unclear about how ideological preoccupation and biases were dealt with Limitations of the study were addressed
Ringwalt, Vincus, Ennett, Hanley, Bowling, Yacoubian, and Rohrbach(2009)	Cross-sectional survey in spring 2005	No cause-effect inference could be drawn from the findings Random samples were selected Data collection procedures were well-designed Descriptive statistics were the main form of analyses Design and statistical analyses were strong Limitations of the study addressed Only quantitative data were collected
Yamaguchi, Johnston, and O'Malley(2003).	Cross-sectional national survey from 1998 to 2001	No cause-effect inference could be drawn from the findings Large sample size in different samples Hierarchical linear models were examined Psychometric properties of the instruments not clear Background confounding factors not properly examined Limitations of the study discussed Only quantitative data were collected
What Works Clearinghouse (2008, May)	Review of Goldberg et al.'s (2007) study	Sample attrition problem leading to bias Non-completion of questionnaires leading to bias Initial differences between the experimental and control groups might create confounding The conclusion of the study does not conform to What Works Clearinghouse standards

What We Found

Several observations can be highlighted from the review. First, not many studies have been conducted to examine the effectiveness of school drug testing since its introduction. With particular reference to the Chinese culture, no study has been conducted in different Chinese contexts. Second, most of the empirical studies were cross-sectional in nature (e.g., surveys and qualitative interviews) and not many experimental studies have been conducted. Third, while there are studies supporting school drug testing (see Table 2), there are also studies not supporting the scheme (see Table 3). Fourth, as shown in Table 4, quality of the existing studies was generally not high, therefore creating doubts regarding their conclusions on the effectiveness of drug test. Basically, there were few well-designed quantitative studies and well-crafted qualitative evaluation studies in the field.

Discussion

Despite the heightened public concern regarding school drug testing and its controversial nature, the number of empirical studies examining the effectiveness of drug test in the school context is surprisingly few. From the perspective of evidence-based practice, research studies play an indispensable role in clarifying the effectiveness of school drug testing and providing support for the policy. As Chinese people constitute roughly one-fifth of the world's population, the absence of school drug testing research is definitely undesirable, particularly in view of the fact that mandatory drug test is legally acceptable in mainland China. In particular, research on school drug testing is indispensable when voluntary school drug testing was implemented in Tai Po district of Hong Kong on a trial basis in 2008.

The present review shows that there are mixed findings on the effectiveness of school drug testing. It should be pointed out that while there are findings showing that drug test had no positive effect, there are findings supporting the effectiveness of school drug testing. This picture is clearly shown in the study of Goldberg et al.(7), one of the few prospective trials in the field. As pointed out by Goldberg et al.(7), "although these findings may differ in other schools or regions of the United Sates, this study *lends credence to some DAT deterrent effects*, especially for past year use for drugs, at two time points, and for drugs and alcohol at two time points. However, because *some substance abuse mediators appeared to worsen and past month substance use never changed*, more research should be performed to assess the policy of drug and alcohol testing's overall effects" (p. 428). The editorial of Journal of Adolescent Health (8) similarly pointed out that "although we might hope that the present study by Goldberg would help to end the national debate, this hope is unlikely to be realized on the basis of this report, which includes ample 'evidence' to fuel the fire on both sides" (p. 419).

As far as the quality of the studies under review is concerned, the review shows that the quality of the existing studies was not high. In addition, it is noteworthy that the findings in the studies under review cannot give a definitive answer to the question of whether school drug testing is effective. For example, although a large sample size was used in the study of Yamaguchi, Johnston, and O'Malley (9), the limitation of the study was that "because of the cross-sectional design of the study, one cannot make definitive causal interpretations regarding effects of drug testing; only a panel design in a randomized or natural experiment can do so. Perhaps schools that instituted drug testing initially had higher use, and drug testing reduced those levels to levels similar to those at other schools" (p. 164) and "this study explored the association between student drug use and drug-testing policies in schools. While lack of evidence for the effectiveness of drug testing is not definitive, results suggest that drug testing in schools may not provide a panacea for reducing student drug use that some (including some on the Supreme Court) had hoped" (p. 164). Unfortunately, probably because of the large sample involved, this study has commonly been taken as evidence against school drug testing.

Obviously, the sustainability of school drug testing depends principally on the amount and quality of research evidence supporting its value and effectiveness. There are two lines of evaluation research that should be done in future. First, quantitative research utilizing experimental designs should be conducted. However, there are at least six issues that should be addressed in experimental studies. First, selection bias (pre-group differences) may confound the results. Studies utilizing pre-experimental designs such as the one conducted by Yamaguchi et al. (9) are particularly vulnerable to this threat. Second, it is noteworthy that drug test scheme will heighten other schools' sensitivity about drug prevention which may minimize the treatment effect in the experimental groups. Third, it is possible that experimental schools may setup anti-drug measures in schools which would eventually exaggerate the treatment effect of school drug testing. Fourth, political and community responses to drug test scheme may influence student attitudes before, during, and after the implementation process. Fifth, the choice of outcome measures and honest disclosure of substance abuse behavior will definitely affect the evaluation outcomes. Sixth, as adolescent substance abuse may have a low base rate in places like Hong Kong, it may be difficult to detect real differences between the experimental group and control group unless very large sample sizes and sensitive measures are used. Finally, researchers have to carefully consider whether "blinding" can be feasibly and meaningfully carried out in related experimental studies.

The second line of research is qualitative evaluation studies. Besides those qualitative findings reported in academic journals (see Tables 2 and 3), there are numerous qualitative accounts of the value and problems of school drug testing. For example, while a high school principal pointed out that "the committee worked very hard to provide a tool which would have a positive effect on our students. The extremely low number of positive tests indicates the program is worth the cost" (10), Knight and Levy (11) warned that "let us not rush to accept the illusory view that drug testing in schools is the silver bullet for the prevention of youth substance abuse...While (dug tests) are increasing in popularity, their efficacy is unproven and they are associated with significant technical concerns".

When researchers conduct qualitative evaluation of school drug testing, it is important to pay particular attention to the rigor of the studies. Shek, Tang, and Han (12) pointed out that there are 12 principles that should be upheld in qualitative evaluation studies. These included: a) statement of the philosophical base of the study; b) justifications for the number and nature of the participants of the study; c) detailed description of data collection procedures; d) discussion of biases in the study; e) description of steps taken to guard against biases or arguments that biases should and/or could not be eliminated; f) pay attention to reliability issues; g) considering out triangulation strategies; h) use of peer checking and member checking; i) use of audit trails; j) examination of alternative explanations; k) accounting for negative evidence; and l) examination of limitations of the study. Obviously, methodological rigor of future qualitative evaluation studies in this field can be strengthened by upholding these principles.

Adopting a balanced perspective, school testing scheme may not be a panacea for adolescent substance abuse. In the long run, effort should be made to integrate school drug test with other preventive measures, such as preventive drug education and positive youth development (13-16) to help young people to stay away from drugs. Fundamentally, it is important to take an evidence-based approach to evaluate the strategies to tackle adolescent substance abuse, including the school drug testing scheme.

ACKNOWLEDGMENTS

The preparation for this paper was financially supported by The Hong Kong Jockey Club Charities Trust.

APPENDIX 1: STUDIES UNDER REVIEW

Barrington K. Voluntary, randomized, student drug-testing: impact in a rural, low-income, community. *J. Alcohol Drug Educ.* 2008;52(1):47-66.
Coombs RH, Coombs CJ. The impact of drug testing on the morale and well-being of mandatory participants. *Int. J. Addict.* 1991;26(9):981-92.
Coombs RH, Ryan FJ. Drug testing effectiveness in identifying and preventing drug use. *Am. J. Drug Alcohol Abuse* 1990;16:173-84.
DuPont RL, Campbell TG, Mazza JJ. *Report of a preliminary study: Elements of a successful school-based student drug testing program.* United States: Institute for Behavior and Health, 2002.
Evans GD, Reader S, Liss HJ, Wiens BA, Roy A. Implementation of an aggressive random drug-testing policy in a rural school district: student attitudes regarding program fairness and effectiveness. *J. Sch. Health* 2006;76(9):452-8.
Evans-Whipp TJ, Bond L, Toumbourou JW, Catalano RF. School, parent, and student perspectives of school drug policies. *J. Sch. Health* 2007;77(3):138-46.
Goldberg L, Elliot DL, MacKinnon DP, Moe E, Kuehl KS, Nohre L, et al. Drug testing athletes to prevent substance abuse: background and pilot study results of the SATURN study. *J. Adolesc. Health* 2003;32(1):16-25.
Goldberg L, Elliot DL, MacKinnon DP, Moe EL, Kuehl KS, Yoon M, et al. Outcomes of a prospective trial of student-athlete drug testing: the student athlete testing using random notification (SATURN) study. *J. Adolesc. Health* 2007;41(5):421-9.
Mason K. *Drug testing in schools: Attitudes of high school students.* PhD thesis, University of New Orleans, 2003.
McKinney JR. *The effectiveness and legality of random drug testing policies.* United States: Student Drug-testing Coalition, 2002.
McKinney JR. *The effectiveness of random drug testing programs: A statewide follow-up study.* United States: Student Drug-testing Coalition, 2003.
McKinney JR. *Effectiveness of student random drug-testing programs.* United States: Student Drug-testing Coalition, 2005.
Ringwalt C, Vincus AA, Ennett ST, Hanley S, Bowling JM, Yacoubian GS, et al. Responses to positive results from suspicion-less random drug tests in United States public school districts. *J. Sch. Health* 2009;79(4):177-83.
What Works Clearinghouse. WWC quick review of the article "Outcomes of a prospective trial of student-athlete drug testing: the student athlete testing using random notification (SATURN) study". United States: Institute of Education Science, Department of

Education, 2008. Accessed 2011 Feb 11. Available at:http://www.ies.ed.gov/ncee/wwc/ publications/ quickreviews/Saturn/index.asp.

Yamaguchi R, Johnston LD, O'Malley PM. Relationship between student illicit drug use and school drug-testing policies. *J. Sch. Health* 2003;73(4):159-64.

REFERENCES

[1] Shek DTL. Tackling adolescent substance abuse in Hong Kong: where we should go and should not go?ScientificWorld Journal 2007;7:2021-30.

[2] Shek DTL. International conference on tackling drug abuse: Conference proceedings. Hong Kong: Narcotics Division, Security Bureau, Government of Hong Kong Special Administrative Region, 2006.

[3] Johnston LD, O'Malley PM, Bachman JG, Schulenberg JE. Monitoring the future:National survey results on drug use, 1975-2008. Vol I: secondary school students(NIH Publication No. 09-7402). Bethesda, MD: National Instititute on Drug Abuse, 2009.

[4] Office of Applied Studies, Substance Abuse and Mental Health Services Administration, U.S. Department of Health and Human Services. Results from the 2008national survey on drug use and health: National findings. Accessed 2011 Feb 11. Available at:http://www.oas.samhsa.gov/ nsduh/2k8nsduh/2k8Results.cfm#2.2.

[5] Office of National Drug Control Policy. What you need to know about starting a student drug-testing program. Washington, DC: Office of National Drug Control Policy, Drug Policy Information Clearing House, 2004: v-vi, 18-9.

[6] Roche AM, Bywood P, Pidd K, Freeman T, Steenson T. Drug testing in Australian schools: policy implications and considerations of punitive, deterrence and/or prevention measures. Int. J. Drug Policy 2009;20(6):521-8.

[7] Goldberg L, Elliot DL, MacKinnon DP, Moe EL, Kuehl KS, Yoon M, et al. Outcomes of a prospective trial of student-athlete drug testing: the student athlete testing using random notification (SATURN) study. J. Adolesc. Health 2007;41(5):421-9.

[8] Knight JR, Levy S. Editorial: the national debate on drug testing in schools. J. Adolesc. Health 2007;41:419-20.

[9] Yamaguchi R, Johnston LD, O'Malley PM. Relationship between student illicit drug use and school drug-testing policies. J. Sch. Health 2003;73(4):159-64.

[10] Edwards CE. Student random drug-testing prevention programs: do these programs work? Drug Watch International 2008. Accessed 2011 Feb 11. Available at: http://www.drugwatch.org/reports/ DWISDT.pdf.

[11] Kern J, Gunja F, Cox A, Rosenbaum M, Appel J, Verma A. Making sense of student drug testing: why educators are saying no, 2nd ed. Drug Policy Alliance 2006. Accessed 2011 Feb 11. Available at: http://www.drugpolicy.org/docUploads/drug_testing_ booklet.pdf.

[12] Shek DTL, Tang V, Han XY. Evaluation of evaluation studies utilizing qualitative research methods in the social work literature (1990-2003): evidence that constitutes a wakeup call. Res. Soc. Work Pract.2005;15:180-94.

[13] Shek DTL, Ng CSM. Subjective outcome evaluation of the Project P.A.T.H.S. (Secondary 2 Program): views of the program participants. ScientificWorld Journal 2009;9:1012-22.

[14] Shek DTL, Sun RCF, Tang CYP. Experimental implementation of the Secondary 3 Program of Project P.A.T.H.S.: observations based on the co-walker scheme.ScientificWorld Journal 2009;9:1003-11.

[15] Shek DTL, Ma HK, Sun RCF. Interim evaluation of the Tier 1 Program (Secondary 1 Curriculum) of the Project P.A.T.H.S.: first year of the Full Implementation Phase. ScientificWorld Journal2008;8:47-60.

[16] Shek DTL. Special issue: evaluation of Project P.A.T.H.S. in Hong Kong. Scientific World Journal2008;8:1-94.

Section One: Project Astro

In: Drug Abuse in Hong Kong
Editors: D Shek, R Sun and J Merrick

ISBN: 978-1-61324-491-3
©2012 Nova Science Publishers, Inc.

Chapter 4

THE PROJECT ASTRO AND DRUG PREVENTION FOR HIGH-RISK YOUTHS IN HONG KONG

Chiu-Wan Lam[1,a] and Daniel TL Shek [,a,b,c,d,e]

[a]Department of Applied Social Sciences,
The Hong Kong Polytechnic University, Hong Kong, PRC
[b]Public Policy Research Institute,
The Hong Kong Polytechnic University, Hong Kong, PRC
[c]East China Normal University, Shanghai, PRC
[d]Kiang Wu Nursing College of Macau, Macau, PRC
[e]Division of Adolescent Medicine, Department of Pediatrics,
Kentucky Children's Hospital, University of Kentucky,
College of Medicine, Lexington, Kentucky, US

ABSTRACT

Conscious of the need to develop an indigenous drug prevention program that is evidence-based and systematic, the Project Astro was designed in Hong Kong focusing on comprehensive strategies that target early risk factors and that strengthen protective factors in adolescence. It

---

[1]Correspondence: Chiu-Wan Lam, MSW, PhD, Department of Applied Social Sciences, The Hong Kong Polytechnic University, Hunghom, Hong Kong. E-mail: sscwlam@polyu.edu.hk.

consisted of three psychosocial primary prevention programs conducted in structured group session. A three-year longitudinal study using a non-equivalent group design was carried out to evaluate the project. Taken as a whole, the findings showed that the participants in the experimental group generally performed better than the control group in terms of social skills, knowledge of drugs, refusal skills, attitudes towards drugs, and the behavioral intention to avoid drug abuse. The present study provides support for the effectiveness of the Project Astro in Hong Kong.

INTRODUCTION

There is a dearth of systematic and documented drug prevention programs in Hong Kong(1,2). In fact, no vigorous evaluation studies exist with a longitudinal design utilizing data from different sources in Chinese communities. As an attempt to fill this gap, this paper introduces the Project Astro and the methods adopted to evaluate the programs.

Recent approaches to drug prevention have focused on comprehensive strategies that target early risk factors and strengthen protective factors in adolescence. Risk factors include poor social skills, low self-esteem, adverse family environment, negative peer influence, poor school performance, and delinquent behaviors (3). With these concerns in mind, Hawkins, Catalano, and Miller (4) proposed that effective drug prevention strategies include parenting skills training, social competence abilities training, and youth involvement in alternative activities. This risk-focused approach aims at reducing the effects of the known antecedents of adolescent drug abuse and cultivating protective factors in high-risk youths. In a similar vein, McNeal and Hansen (5) also identified four key mediators of adolescent drug use: commitment not to use drugs, lifestyle incompatibility with drug use, beliefs about the consequences of drug use, and normative beliefs such as peer beliefs and endorsement of drug use. Since effective drug prevention work should seek to reduce adolescents' vulnerability to unfavorable environmental factors and eliminate environmental influences that induce drug use (6), an increasing emphasis has been placed on the use of structured intervention programs in drug prevention for young people, such as the "SMART" program (7,8), "Drug Abuse Resistance and Education" (DARE) (9,10), and "Project STAR" (11).

Conscious of the need to develop an indigenous drug prevention program that is evidence-based, systematic, and conceptually sound, the "Astro" (Anti Substance Tobacco Refusal Operation) project was designed by this research team for high-risk youths in Hong Kong. A "high-risk youth" was defined as an adolescent who fulfilled any two or more of the following criteria: a) attending a school of low academic standard; b) exhibition of conduct problems, such as truancy; c) a dropout from school and/or unemployed; d) drug use experience, particularly abuse of stimulants and/or polydrugs; e) frequent smoking. It was expected that this drug prevention program would: a) increase the participants' knowledge about drugs and sex; b) improve their attitudes toward substance abuse and sex; c) strengthen their ability to refuse drugs and early sex;and d) reduce their actual usage of drugs and engagement in sex.

The Project Astro consisted of three psychosocial primary prevention programs conducted in structured group sessions for youths (i.e., Astro Kids, aged 10 to 13; Astro Teens, aged 13 to 16; and Astro Leaders). Ideally, an adolescent would complete all the programs, but each program had its own independent functions. The goals of the Project Astro were to increase the participants' knowledge about drugs, help them develop proper attitudes toward substance abuse, strengthen their ability to refuse drugs, and reduce the participants' usage of drugs. Apart from providing drug information, the programs also taught young people a broad range of social and personal competence skills to resist peer and other social pressures.

Each program consists of 10 to 12 sessions, which cover the following areas: stress and stress management, family relationships, knowledge of gateway drugs (i.e., cigarettes and alcohol), psychotropic drugs (i.e., "ice", ketamine, marijuana, and ecstasy) and sex, peer influence, self-understanding, and refusal skills.

The programs were organized in youth centers, primary and secondary schools. A complete set of manuals for program delivery and evaluation were prepared (12). Training sessions for parents, social workers, and community leaders were held as follows:

Astro Kids program

The total number of groups in the Astro Kids program was 13, with 139 experimental subjects and 213 control subjects (N=352). The Astro Kids program consists of 10 sessions, with some sessions conducted at day or overnight camps. The contents of the program include: stress and stress management, family relationships, knowledge about gateway drugs, psychotropic drugs and sex, peer influence, stress from media, self-understanding, and refusal skills.

Astro Teens program

The total number of groups in the Astro Teens program was 20, with 217 experimental subjects and 201 control subjects (N=418). The Astro Teens program consists of 10 to 12 sessions, with some sessions conducted at day or overnight camps. The contents of the program include: stress and stress management, decision-making, knowledge about gateway drugs, psychotropic drugs and sex, peer influence, self-esteem, and refusal skills.

Astro Leaders Program

The total number of groups in the Astro Leaders program was 11, with 92 experimental subjects. As the Astro Leaders graduated from the Astro Teens program, the pre-post assessments of Astro Leaders and their control group were based on the pre-post assessments when they were in the program. The Astro Leaders program consisted of three group sessions on sensitivity and leadership training as well as one community involvement project (e.g., a hip hop dance show, game stalls on Parents' Day for reinforcing parent-child bonding, visits to the elderly, volunteer services for spastic children, and an adventure-based counseling camp for Astro Teens members).

Parents' program (FAN Club)

The total number of FAN Club activities was 14, with 197 participants. The activities included workshops, group discussions, talks, day camps, and a parent-child carnival. The focus of the activities included parent-child communication, conflict resolution, parental roles in youth drug prevention, and parent-child bonding.

Training for workers

Whole-day training workshops were held for workers to explain the rationale, research methodology, design of the project, and the role expectations of group leaders. Sessions for workers to share their experiences and offer feedback on the project were also arranged. A total of 66 workers participated in these training activities.

Activities for community leaders

Training workshops and sharing sessions were held for 51 community leaders (such as district board members, police, and school principals), during which they discussed the role of the community in youth drug prevention.

Astro Club

The Astro Club was formed to provide healthy activities for its members, such as adventure-based counseling sessions, visits to the drug rehabilitation center, and exhibition and game stalls to promote drug prevention. A total of 323 people participated in the activities.

Taking into account the merits of different program evaluation approaches (13,14), a design that utilized different evaluation strategies and facilitated the triangulation of different kinds of data was adopted in this research, including: a) a quasi-experimental design study based on objective outcome indicators; b) subjective outcome evaluation based on the responses of social workers and participants; c) qualitative evaluation based on in-depth interviews with participants, teachers, and social workers who had assisted in running the programs; and d) evaluation based on repertory grid tests of the participants that assessed their self-identity systems before and after joining the program.

OUR STUDY

Evaluation design and participants

A three-year longitudinal study adopting a quasi-experimental design was adopted in this project for the program evaluation. Since it was difficult to randomly assign the subjects in the experimental and control groups, a nonequivalent group design was adopted. The participants were asked to complete self-administered questionnaires at pretest (before the first session of the program) and posttest 1 (within two weeks after the program). Six months later, some of the participants followed up with the same questionnaire (posttest 2). The numbers of respondents in the experimental and control groups are presented in Table 1. It should be noted that 40 participants (about 5% of all participants) left the Astro program and did not complete the first posttest. Analyses of the differences between completers

Table 1. Number of respondents in the experimental and control groups, and distribution of respondents in the drug group and the non-drug group

	Astro Kids			Astro Teens			Drug group		Non-drug group	
	Pretest	Post1	Post2	Pretest	Post1	Post2	N	%*	N	%*
Experimental	139	134	85	217	200	104	255	35%	79	11%
Control	213	203	62	201	193	88	248	34%	148	20%
Total	352	337[a]	147	418	393[b]	192	503[c]	69%	227[d]	31%

*Percentage of total number of participants in the Posttest 1 (N=730).
(a + b)or (c + d) = 730 (i.e., total number of participants in the posttest).

and noncompleters suggested that it is unlikely that the findings were significantly affected by sample attrition. The details can be seen in Table 1.

Instruments

At the pretest, posttest 1 and 2 sessions (within two weeks and six months after they had accomplished the programs respectively), the participants were invited to complete a self-administered questionnaire that included different measures of substance abuse and psychosocial adjustment. For the measures of social skills and substance abuse, they were translated and adapted from the evaluation questionnaire originally constructed by St. Pierre and Kaltreider (15). Other scales were developed by the research team except the seventh one:

1. *Social Skills Scale*: This scale assessed the perceived social skills of the respondents who were asked to rate their ability to perform some social behaviors (e.g., speaking to strangers).The respondent was asked to rate his/her ability to perform some social behavior on a 4-point scale ("Very Unable", "Unable", "Able", "Very Able"). A higher total score indicates a higher level of social skills in the scale.
2. *Attitude (All drugs) Scale*: Indicators of attitudes to psychotropic drugs and "all drugs" were developed. A total of 51 items were developed to assess the respondents' attitudes to smoking (6 items), drinking (8 items), marijuana (6 items), heroin (7 items), ecstasy (6 items), ketamine (7 items), methylamphetamine ("ice", 7 items), and sex (4 items). The respondents were asked to respond to the attitudinal statements on a 4-pont scale ("Strongly Disagree", "Disagree", "Agree", "Strongly Agree"). By combining the scores related to smoking and drinking (14

items), a measure of attitude to gateway drugs was developed. Similarly, by adding items in the relevant measures, indicators of attitudes to psychotropic drugs and all drugs were developed. A total of 11 measures of attitudes to substance abuse and sex were used in this study. Lower scale scores indicate perceptions of fewer benefits of taking drug or engaging in sexual behavior.

3. *Refusal Scale*: Several 2-item scales were developed to assess the participants' abilities of refusing alcohol, smoking, marijuana, heroin, ecstasy, ketamine, and methylamphetamine ("ice"). The respondents were asked to respond whether they would find it difficult to refuse the above substances given by their friends on a 5-point scale (e.g., "Very Difficult to Refuse", "Slightly Difficult to Refuse", "Don't Know", "Slightly Easy to Refuse", "Very Easy to Refuse"). By combining items on alcohol and smoking, a measure of refusal skills on gateway drugs was formed (4 items). Similarly, by adding up the scores of the relevant measures, indicators of refusal skills regarding psychotropic drugs and all drugs were developed. A total of 11 measures of refusal skills on substance abuse and sex were used in this study. A higher scale score indicates a higher level of perceived ability to refuse the drug.

4. *Usage Scale*: Four scales were developed to measure the respondent's use of drugs (e.g., alcohol, smoking, heroin) and engagement in sexual behavior with reference to four time points: last 7 days, last 30 days, last 3 months, and ever. There are 9 items in each section and 11 measures for each time frame. A higher score refers to a higher level of substance abuse or sexual behavior in this section.

5. *Behavioral Intention Scale*: A total of 8 items were developed to assess whether the respondent would engage in substance abuse and sexual behavior in the next two years. For each item, the respondent was requested to respond to a 4-point scale ("Definitely Will", "Probably Will", "Probably Will Not", "Definitely Will Not"). There are 11 measures derived from the items in this section. A higher score refers to a lower behavioral intention to take drugs or engage in sexual behavior in the near future.

6. *All Knowledge (drugs and sex) Scale*: A total of 26 items were developed to measure drug knowledge (18 items) and sex knowledge (8 items). For each item, the respondent was asked to respond to a 2-point scale ("True" or "False"). A higher score in these scales refers to a higher level of drug knowledge or sex knowledge.

7. *Chinese Self-Esteem Scale:* The Rosenberg Self-Esteem Scale was designed to assess the self-esteem of high school students (17). The Chinese Rosenberg Self-Esteem Scale was developed by one of the authors and acceptable reliability of this scale has been reported (1,18).

Data analytic strategies

For the assessment of the effects of the intervention, we adopted the analysis of covariance (ANCOVA), which is a widely used strategy to examine the outcome data emerging from a non-equivalent group study. We also observed other researchers' experiences (19-21) and included a number of variables as covariates in the ANCOVA analyses. These covariates included "gender" and the pretest scores of two variables under study, namely, the respondents' psychological well-being (self-esteem and general psychological health) and the tendency towards delinquency. The scale scores of the respondents' drug attitude, behavioral intention toward drugs, refusal, and usage in the "all drugs" category at pretest were also included as covariates in each analysis, because we had found that the experimental and control groups differed in all these aspects at pretest.

After the effects of covariates were controlled, we investigated the effectiveness of the Astro programs by examining the differences in outcome indicators between the experimental and control groups at posttest (assigned as the "Group" variable).

OUR FINDINGS

Analyses of the pretest-posttest 1 data

Several analyses were carried out with reference to different time frames. The first set of analyses was primarily concerned with the results of the participants' data obtained from the pretest and the first posttest (within two weeks after the program) of the Astro Kids and Astro Teens. It was found that the scales had satisfactory coefficients of reliability both in the pretest (M=0.75) and the posttest (M=0.77). It was also found that the experimental and control groups differed in terms of some of the outcome indicators at pretest (Table 2), and the control group had less usage of all kinds of drugs than the experimental group in the last 30 days (T=2.15, p<.05) and three months (T=3.04, p<.01). Hence, the effects of these

Table 2. Differences between experimental group and control group at pretest

Measures	Experimental Group (M)	Control Group (M)	Direction	T	Sig.
Combined Sample (N=730)					
C Behavioral intention (Ecstasy)	3.58	3.71	H	-1.989	*
C Behavioral intention(All drugs)	27.47	27.52	H	-2.450	*
C Behavioral intention (Alcohol)	2.66	3.01	H	-4.288	#
C Behavioral intention (Smoking)	2.95	3.29	H	-3.869	#
C Behavioral intention (Gateway)	5.60	6.30	H	-4.517	#
C Attitude (Ecstasy)	12.20	11.32	L	2.852	**
C Attitude ("Ice")	11.93	11.08	L	2.849	**
C Attitude (Marijuana)	9.41	8.92	L	2.008	*
C Attitude (Psycho drugs)	43.72	40.69	L	3.002	***
C Attitude(All drugs)	70.71	65.58	L	3.409	***
C Attitude (Smoking)	10.18	9.37	L	2.617	**
C Attitude (Gateway)	26.99	24.89	L	3.457	***
C Refusal skills (All drugs)	33.00	34.64	H	-3.002	**
C Delinquency	32.41	27.96	L	4.137	#
C Self-esteem	13.45	13.92	H	-2.420	*

C: Control group is better than experimental group; H: The higher the better; L: The lower the better; #$p<=0.0001$;***$p<=0.001$;**$p<=0.01$;*$p<=0.05$.

preconditions on the dependent variables at posttest needed to be adjusted in the analysis (as shown in Table 2).

The results of the ANCOVA analyses for both groups of respondents of the pretest and posttest 1 data that were statistically significant are presented in Table 3. The scores in Social Skills Scale and All Knowledge (drugs and sex) Scale of the respondents in the experimental group were better than those in the control group in the combined sample. With closer scrutiny, by further dividing the two groups into different samples, we found that the experimental group's attitude towards "ice" was also more positive (i.e., less susceptible to the drug) in the sample of female kids. However, the respondents in the experimental group were worse than their counterparts in the control group if the experimental group's attitudes to substance abuse were examined. This tendency could be seen in the kids' attitudes towards marijuana and smoking. For the male kids, the

Table 3. ANCOVA analyses of the Posttest-1 data for all samples

	Scale	Experimental Group (M)	Control Group (M)	Direction	F value	Sig.
		Combined Sample (N=730)				
E	Social skills	18.24	17.84	H	5.345	*
E	All knowledge (Drugs & sex)	19.00	18.60	H	3.936	*
C	Attitude (Smoking)	12.02	11.59	L	5.284	*
		Male Sample (N=422)				
C	Attitude (Smoking)	12.09	11.49	L	5.535	*
		Female Sample (N=308)				
C	Behav. intention (Smoking)	2.93	3.15	H	5.23	*
		Kids Sample (N=337)				
C	Attitude (Marijuana)	9.05	8.41	L	5.631	*
C	Attitude (Smoking)	11.16	10.43	L	7.997	**
		Male Kids Sample (N=208)				
C	Attitude (Ecstasy)	9.53	8.73	L	4.684	*
C	Attitude (Marijuana)	9.38	8.41	L	7.858	**
C	Attitude (All drugs)	78.23	72.17	L	5.189	*
C	Attitude (Smoking)	11.65	10.46	L	11.836	***
		Female Kids Sample (N=129)				
E	Attitude ("Ice")	9.84	10.95	L	3.796	*

C: Control group is better than experimental group; E: Experimental group is better than control group; H: The higher the better; L: The lower the better; ***$p<=0.001$; **$p<=0.01$; *$p<=0.05$.

experimental group's attitudes towards ecstasy, marijuana, "all drugs" and smoking were also poorer at posttest.

The respondents were further divided into a "drug group" and a "non-drug group" according to their experiences of abusing drugs or the absence of such behavior in the second stage of analysis of the effects of the programs. It was found that, of the 17 statistically significant findings summarized in Table 4, nine were of a positive direction. For the drug group, the social skills of the experimental group were better than those of the control group for the samples of female respondents and kids. Moreover, the evidence suggested that the experimental group's knowledge of drugs and sex (All knowledge) was better than that of the control group for the samples of female respondents and female teens. In addition, the kids in the experimental group had weaker intention to abuse heroin than did the corresponding sample in the control group. This was also found for the sample of male kids in regard to their intention to abuse ecstasy, ketamine, and heroin, and in regard to the "all drugs" variable. On the other hand, refusal skills were observed to be higher in the control group than in the experimental group for male respondents (in regard to ketamine and alcohol),

Table 4. ANCOVA analyses of the Posttest-1 data for the drug group

	Scale	Experimental Group (M)	Control Group (M)	Direction	F value	Sig.
		Male Sample (N=293)				
C	Refusal skills (Ketamine)	8.07	8.48	H	5.45	*
C	Refusal skills (Alcohol)	6.92	7.38	H	4.193	*
		Female Sample (N=210)				
E	Social skills	18.28	17.79	H	3.968	*
E	All knowledge	19.56	18.90	H	3.665	*
		Female Teens Sample (N=157)				
E	All knowledge	19.70	18.81	H	4.316	*
		Kids Sample (N=168)				
E	Social Skills	18.49	17.67	H	4.739	*
E	Behavioral intention (Heroin)	3.70	3.39	H	4.649	*
C	Refusal skills (Ecstasy)	8.09	8.54	H	3.881	*
C	Refusal skills (Ketamine)	8.14	8.57	H	3.935	*
C	Refusal skills(Alcohol)	7.09	7.63	H	3.839	*
		Male Kids Sample (N=115)				
E	Behavioral intention (Ecstasy)	3.63	3.22	H	4.916	*
E	Behavioral intention (Ketamine)	3.61	3.25	H	4.148	*
E	Behavioral intention (Heroin)	3.74	3.27	H	7.085	**
E	Behavioral intention (All drugs)	23.64	21.39	H	3.959	*
C	Attitude (Marijuana)	10.19	9.01	L	5.715	*
C	Attitude (Smoking)	12.46	11.51	L	4.136	*
		Female Kids Sample (N=53)				
C	Refusal skills ("Ice")	8.36	9.05	H	4.037	*

C: Control group is better than experimental group; E: Experimental group is better than control group; H: The higher the better; L: The lower the better; **$p<=0.01$; *$p<=0.05$.

female kids (in regard to "ice"), and the samples of kids (in regard to ecstasy, ketamine, and alcohol). The male kids in the control group also had a lower tendency to abuse marijuana than did the experimental group (see Table 4).

For the non-drug group (Table 5), the analyses of posttest 1 data showed that 15 of the 20 significant findings were positive. The experimental group had higher refusal skills than the control group for the samples of male respondents (in regard to ketamine, "ice", heroin, alcohol and smoking) and male teens (in regard to ecstasy, ketamine, psychotropic substances, and "all drugs"). Knowledge of drugs and sex ("Drug knowledge" and "All knowledge") for the different samples (i.e., male respondents, male teens and male kids) of the experimental group was also better than that of their counterparts in the control group. For the female kids, the experimental group perceived less benefits of abusing psychotropic drugs than the control group did. In contrast, the combined sample and the female respondents

Table 5. ANCOVA analyses of the Posttest-1 data for the non-drug group

	Scale	Experimental Group (M)	Control Group (M)	Direction	F Value	Sig.
		Combined Sample (N=227)				
C	Attitude (Marijuana)	8.78	8.03	L	4.898	*
		Male Sample (N=129)				
E	Refusal skills (Ketamine)	8.92	8.27	H	4.834	*
E	Refusal skills ("Ice")	9.00	8.33	H	5.330	*
E	Refusal skills (Heroin)	9.00	8.43	H	3.953	*
E	Refusal skills (Alcohol)	8.68	7.99	H	3.838	*
E	Refusal skills (Smoking)	8.89	8.36	H	5.065	*
E	Drug knowledge	13.50	12.35	H	8.692	*
E	All knowledge	19.10	17.56	H	9.193	*
		Female Sample (N=98)				
C	Attitude (Marijuana)	9.04	8.02	L	4.631	*
		Male Teens Sample (N=36)				
E	Refusal skills (Ecstasy)	9.31	8.36	H	5.258	*
E	Refusal skills (Ketamine)	9.15	8.15	H	4.549	*
E	Refusal skills (Psycho. drugs)	17.84	15.57	H	4.531	*
E	Refusal skills (All drugs)	30.85	27.17	H	4.437	*
E	Drug knowledge	14.38	12.05	H	9.855	*
E	All knowledge	20.21	17.62	H	5.510	*
		Male Kids Sample (N=93)				
C	Attitude (Alcohol)	14.82	13.43	L	4.765	**
C	Attitude (Smoking)	10.48	9.30	L	5.475	*
C	Behavioral intention (Smoking)	3.62	3.91	H	4.535	**
E	All knowledge	18.70	17.51	H	4.103	*
		Female Kids Sample (N=76)				
E	Attitude (Psycho. drugs)	36.52	37.93	L	5.066	*

C: Control group is better than experimental group; E: Experimental group is better than control group; H: The higher the better; L: The lower the better; **$p<=0.01$; *$p<=0.05$.

in the control group perceived less benefits of abusing marijuana than their counterparts in the experimental group.

Regarding the usage of drugs for all respondents (N=730), it was found that the control group abused less gateway drugs in the last 7 and 30 days among the combined sample and the samples of male, female and kid respondents. However, for the use of heroin, the experimental group had a better record than that of the control group in the combined and teens samples. For the drug group (N=503), there was evidence that among the combined sample, the experimental group had taken less heroin and smoking than the control group did in the last 7 and 30 days. Similar performances were detected for the teens in smoking, and the male

Table 6. Comparison of drug use behavior between the experimental and control groups (Posttest-1 data)

		Groups comparison	7 days F	Sig.	30 days F	Sig.
		All respondents (N=730)				
Combined sample	Heroin	E	5.994	*	0.106	--
	Smoking	C	6.337	*	6.349	*
	All drugs	C	0.913	--	3.988	*
Male sample	Smoking	C	1.334	--	4.296	*
	All drugs	C	0.19	--	4.38	*
Female sample	Gateway	C	5.260	*	3.046	--
	Smoking	C	6.268	*	1.440	--
Teens sample	Heroin	E	8.093	*	0.280	--
Kids sample	Smoking	C	3.889	*	2.862	--
		Drug group (N=503)				
Combined sample	Smoking	E	4.810	*	3.859	*
	Heroin	E	5.071	*	4.852	*
Male sample	Ketamine	E	6.311	*	5.725	*
	Ecstasy	E	3.996	*	3.683	--
	Psycho. drugs	E	5.596	*	5.137	*
Teens sample	Smoking	E	4.310	*	3.167	--
		Non-drug group (N=227)				
Combined sample	Ketamine	E	0.184	--	5.300	*
	Psycho. drugs	E	0.244	--	4.898	*

C: Control group is better than experimental group; E: Experimental group is better than control group; *$p \leq 0.05$.

respondents in the use of ketamine, ecstasy and psychotropic substances. For the non-drug group (N=227), there was also evidence that among the combined sample, the experimental group took ketamine and psychotropic drugs, though less than the control group in the last 30 days. All in all, of the 17 statistically significant findings summarized in Table 6, ten were of a positive direction.

With reference to the analyses of the posttest data obtained six months after our intervention (Tables 3 to 6), it can be concluded that the effectiveness of the Project Astro can be supported.

Analyses of the pretest-posttest 1-posttest 2 data

The findings based on the ANCOVA analyses for the pretest-posttest 1-posttest 2 data are presented in Table 7. Six positive observations could be seen. First, social skills of the participants in the experimental group were better than those of the control group in the Combined, Teens, Kids, Male, Female and Male Kids Samples. Second, drug knowledge in the experimental group was better than that of the control group in the Teens, Male Teens, and Female Teens Samples. Third, the experimental group performed better than the control group in terms behavioral intention to engage in sexual behavior (Kids Sample and Male Kids Sample) and smoking (Male Kids). Fourth, the experimental group perceived fewer benefits of taking "ice" (Kids and Male Samples) and gateway drugs (Female Teens) than did those of the control group. Fifth, the experimental group displayed higher refusal skills than the control group in resisting ecstasy (Kids and Male Kids Samples), "ice" (Kids, Male and Male Kids Samples), sex (Female Kids Sample), marijuana (Combined, Kids and Male Samples), gateway drugs (Kids and Male Kids Samples), and psychotropic drugs (Kids Sample). Finally, the experimental group displayed less sex behavior in the last 30 days and 3 months than did the control group in the Female Sample. However, the control group was better than the experimental group in terms of attitudes to smoking (Kids Sample) and alcohol (Kids and Male Kids Samples). With reference to the 32 significant findings summarized in Table 7, 29 were positive findings.

For the Drug Group (Table 8), the findings showed that social skills in the experimental group were better than those in the control group in the Combined and Male Samples. There was also evidence suggesting that drug knowledge in the experimental group was higher than that of the control group in the Teens and Male Teens Samples. In addition, the experimental group performed better than the control group in terms of behavioral intention to "ice" (Male Teens) and alcohol (Female Teens). Furthermore, the experimental group perceived fewer benefits of abusing ketamine (Male Kids), heroin (Female Teens), marijuana (Teens), gateway drugs (Combined, Teens, Female, and Female Teens Samples), and psychotropic drugs (Female Teens).

Table 7. ANCOVA analyses of the pretest, Post test-1 and Posttest-2 data

		Post 1- Post 2 Mean		Scale Direction	Main effect Between subject factor Group effect		Interaction effect Group x Time	
		Experimental	Control		F	Sig.	F	Sig.
		Combined Sample (N=339)						
E	Social skills	18.06	17.80	H	12.519	#	--	
E	Refusal skills (Marijuana)	8.39	8.28	H	5.751	*	--	

		Post 1- Post 2 Mean		Scale Direction	Main effect Between subject factor Group effect		Interaction effect Group x Time	
		Experimental	Control		F	Sig.	F	Sig.
E	Drug Knowledge	13.74	13.30	H	7.170	**	--	
	Kids Sample (N=147)							
E	Social skills	18.19	17.50	H	6.726	*	--	
E	Behavioral intention (Sex)	3.63	3.57	H	5.273	*	--	
E	Attitude ("Ice")	10.61	10.82	L	4.781	*	--	
E	Refusal skills (Ecstasy)	8.51	8.31	H	4.837	*	--	
E	Refusal skills ("Ice")	8.45	8.31	H	5.641	*	--	
E	Refusal skills (Marijuana)	8.54	8.27	H	4.327	*	--	
E	Refusal skills (Gateway)	7.93	7.67	H	4.479	*	--	
E	Refusal skills (Psycho. drugs)	16.15	15.63	H	4.290	*	--	
C	Attitude (Alcohol)	15.26	14.28	L	4.297	*	--	
C	Attitude (Smoking)	11.09	10.19	L	6.090	*	--	
	Male Sample (N=193)							
E	Social skills	18.17	17.76	H	10.384	**	--	
E	Attitude ("Ice")	11.27	11.28	L	4.857	*	--	
E	Refusal skills ("Ice")	8.52	8.32	H	4.774	*	--	
E	Refusal skills (Marijuana)	8.56	8.26	H	4.330	*	--	
	Female Sample N=146)							
E	Social skills	17.94	17.82	H	--		4.304	#
E	Usage (Sex) – 30days	0.04	0.22	L	6.903	**	--	
E	Usage (Sex) – 3months	0.07	0.24	L	4.029	*	--	
	Male Kids Sample (N=101)							
E	Social skills	18.37	17.12	H	4.976	*	--	
E	Behavioral intention (Sex)	3.62	3.46	H	4.964	*	--	
E	Behavioral intention (Smoking)	3.56	3.46	H	4.918	*	--	
E	Refusal skills (Ecstasy)	8.46	8.07	H	4.599	*	--	
E	Refusal skills ("Ice")	8.41	8.03	H	4.495	*	--	
E	Refusal skills (Gateway)	8.53	8.10	H	--		5.174	#
C	Attitude (Alcohol)	15.68	14.40	L	5.143	*	--	
	Female Kids Sample (N=46)							
E	Refusal skills (Sex)	2.980	2.975	H	5.129	*	--	
	Male Teens Sample (N=92)							
E	Drug knowledge	13.54	13.32	H	8.176	**	--	
	Female Teens Sample (N=100)							
E	Attitude (Gateway)	29.50	29.55	L	6.477	*	--	
E	Drug knowledge	13.85	13.47	H	4.924	*	--	

C: Control group is better than experimental group; E: Experimental group is better than control group; H: The higher the better; L: The lower the better; $p \leq 0.0001$ (#); ** $p \leq 0.01$; * $p \leq 0.05$.

Table 8. ANCOVA analyses of the pretest, Posttest-1 and Posttest-2 data in the Drug Group

	Post 1- Post 2 Mean Experimental	Control	Scale Direction	Main effect btwn subject factorGroup effect F	Sig.	Interaction effect Group x Time F	Sig.
	Combined Sample (N=187)						
E Social skills	18.31	18.00	H	6.819	**	--	
E Attitude (Gateway)	28.58	29.07	L	4.996	*	--	
C Attitude (Marijuana)	9.62	9.42	L	3.988	*	--	
	Teens Sample (N=135)						
E Attitude (Marijuana)	9.61	9.73	L	5.802	*	--	
E Attitude (Gateway)	30.05	30.94	L	8.264	**	--	
E Drug knowledge	13.74	13.20	H	7.293	**	--	
	Kids Sample (N=51)						
C Attitude (Ketamine)	11.15	10.83	L	--		8.602	**
C Attitude (Ecstasy)	9.49	8.10	L	4.759	*	--	
	Male Sample (N=100)						
E Social skills	18.30	17.92	H	6.253	*	--	
	Female Sample (N=87)						
E Attitude (Gateway)	29.50	29.80	L	4.400	*	--	
E Usage (Sex) – 7days	0.98	2.31	L	7.168	**	--	
E Usage (Sex) – 30days	1.00	2.12	L	5.970	*	--	
E Usage (Sex) – 3months	1.00	2.13	L	5.606	*	--	
	Male Kids Sample (N=37)						
E Attitude (Ketamine)	11.51	11.57	L	--		5.221	*
C Attitude (Alcohol)	17.00	15.08	L	5.145	*	--	
	Female Kids Sample (N=14)						
E Refusal skills(Ecstasy)	9.59	7.55	H	7.550	*	--	
E Refusal skills (Ketamine)	9.56	7.51	H	7.932	*	--	
E Refusal skills("Ice")	9.49	7.60	H	7.766	*	--	
E Refusal skills (Marijuana)	9.73	7.36	H	10.082	*	--	
E Refusal skills (Heroin)	9.71	7.56	H	10.046	*	--	
	Male Teens Sample (N=62)						
E Behavioral intention ("Ice")	3.76	3.59	H	5.046	*	--	
E Drug knowledge	13.61	13.01	H	5.044	*	--	
	Female Teens Sample (N=73)						
E Behavioral intention (Alcohol)	2.04	1.90	H	5.975	*	--	
E Attitude (Heroin)	11.43	11.55	L	4.278	*	--	
E Attitude (Gateway)	30.82	31.56	L	8.444	**	--	
E Attitude (PS)	46.11	46.35	L	5.544	*	--	
C Attitude (Marijuana)	10.18	10.00	L	4.748	*	--	
E Usage (Sex) – 7days	1.17	2.50	L	6.579	*	--	
E Usage (Sex) – 30days	1.11	2.25	L	5.818	*	--	
E Usage (Sex) – 3months	1.15	2.31	L	5.600	*	--	

C: Control group is better than experimental group; E: Experimental group is better than control group; H: The higher the better; L: The lower the better; **$p<=0.01$; *$p<=0.05$.

Table 9. ANCOVA analyses of the pretest, Posttest-1 and Posttest-2 data in the Non-Drug Group

		Post 1- Post 2 Mean		ScaleDirection	Main effect Between subject factor Group effect		Interaction effect Group x Time	
		Experimental	Control		F	Sig.	F	Sig.
		Combined Sample (N=152)						
E	Social skills	17.690	17.629	H	5.666	*	--	
E	Refusal skills (Ecstasy)	8.502	8.483	H	7.419	**	--	
E	Refusal skills (Ketamine)	8.519	8.448	H	4.431	*	--	
E	Refusal skills ("Ice")	8.495	8.477	H	9.335	**	--	
E	Refusal skills (Alcohol)	8.182	8.093	H	8.142	**	--	
C	Behavioral intention (Psycho. drugs)	15.17	15.24	H	4.524	*	--	
		Teens Sample (N=56)						
C	Social skills	16.824	17.627	H	--		10.289	**
		Kids Sample (N=96)						
E	Social skills	18.158	17.628	H	4.911	*	--	
E	Refusal skills (Ecstasy)	8.606	8.458	H	5.847	*	--	
E	Refusal skills ("Ice")	8.507	8.491	H	7.563	**	--	
E	Refusal skills (Alcohol)	8.373	8.366	H	6.535	*	--	
E	Refusal skills (Smoking)	8.582	8.324	H	4.414	*	--	
E	Refusal skills (Marijuana)	8.602	8.488	H	5.841	*	--	
E	Refusal skills (Gateway)	7.969	7.790	H	4.340	*	--	
C	Refusal skills (Sex)	2.799	3.104	H	7.439	**	--	
		Male Sample (N=93)						
E	Social skills	17.899	17.726	H	4.740	*	--	
E	Refusal skills (Ketamine)	8.756	8.217	H	4.159	*	--	
E	Refusal skills ("Ice")	8.655	8.276	H	6.032	*	--	

Table 9. (Continued)

		Post 1- Post 2 Mean		Scale Direction	Main effect Between subject factor Group effect		Interaction effect Group x Time	
		Experimental	Control		F	Sig.	F	Sig.
E	Refusal skills (Alcohol)	8.429	7.877	H	6.020	*	--	
E	Refusal skills (Marijuana)	8.748	8.301	H	5.639	*	--	
E	Sex knowledge	5.960	5.378	H	4.045	*	--	
C	Usage (Gateway) – 30days	2.17	1.59	L	4.205	*	--	
		Female Sample (N=59)						
E	Usage (Alcohol) – 30days	1.12	1.54	L	5.797	*	--	
E	Usage (Alcohol) – 3months	1.10	1.53	L	6.583	*	--	
E	Usage (Gateway) – 30days	1.81	2.56	L	4.784	*	--	
C	Social skills	17.338	17.561	H	--		4.681	*
C	Behavioral intention (Ketamine)	3.558	3.710	H	--		4.330	*
C	Refusal skills (Heroin)	8.253	8.952	H	4.459	*	--	
		Male Kids Sample (N=64)						
E	Behavioral intention (Ketamine)	3.75	3.49	H	5.235	*	--	
E	Behavioral intention (Sex)	3.68	3.36	H	4.54	*	--	
E	Behavioral intention (Alcohol)	3.58	3.18	H	4.86	*	--	
E	Behavioral intention (Smoking)	3.62	3.43	H	9.164	**	--	
E	Behavioral intention (Psycho. drugs)	15.01	13.89	H	4.36	*	--	
E	Refusal skills (Ecstasy)	8.436	8.434	H	6.387	*	--	
E	Refusal skills (Ketamine)	8.78	8.06	H	5.958	*	--	
E	Refusal skills ("Ice")	8.66	8.08	H	6.047	*	--	
E	Refusal skills (Heroin)	8.75	8.21	H	5.477	*	--	

		Post 1- Post 2 Mean		Scale Direction	Main effect Between subject factor Group effect		Interaction effect Group x Time	
		Experimental	Control		F	Sig.	F	Sig.
E	Refusal skills (Marijuana)	8.78	8.12	H	8.435	**	--	
E	Refusal skills (Alcohol)	8.62	8.14	H	4.207	*	--	
E	Refusal skills (Smoking)	8.81	8.04	H	7.96	**	--	
E	Usage (Smoking) – 7days	0.46	0.70	L	11.376	**	--	
E	Usage (Smoking) – 3months	0.48	0.63	L	6.456	*	--	
C	Attitude (Psycho. drugs)	55.01	53.89	L	4.83	*	--	
C	Refusal skills (Sex)	2.70	3.09	H	7.193	**	--	
	Female Kids Sample (N=32)							
E	Refusal skills (Psycho. drugs)	16.98	15.72	H	7.109	*	--	
E	Usage (Alcohol) – 3months	1.10	1.31	L	4.879	*	--	
E	Usage (Gateway) – 3months	1.59	1.88	L	5.672	*	--	
	Male Teens Sample (N=29)							
E	Attitude ("Ice")	11.444	11.703	L	6.298	*	--	
E	Refusal skills ("Ice")	8.852	8.516	H	--		5.558	*
E	Refusal skills (Marijuana)	8.854	8.513	H	--		6.922	*
	Female Teens Sample (N=27)							
E	Social skills	16.979	16.375	H	--		8.105	**
E	Drug knowledge	14.037	13.268	H	--		5.324	*

Notes:
i. In Male Kids analysis, "All Drugs" and "Existential Well-Being" were excluded in the covariates.
ii. C: Control group is better than experimental group; E: Experimental group is better than control group; H: The higher the better; L: The lower the better; **$p<=0.01$; *$p<=0.05$.

Finally, the experimental group displayed higher levels of refusal skills than did the control group in the areas of ecstasy, ketamine, "ice", heroin, and marijuana in the Female Kids Sample. In terms of usage of drugs and sex, there is evidence showing that the experimental group engaged in less sexual behavior than the control group did in the Female Sample and Female Teens Sample. However, some negative findings in the attitudes towards substance abuse were found in the Combined, Kids, Male Kids, and Female Teens Samples. Out of 30 significant findings presented in Table 8, 25 findings were positive.

For the Non-Drug Group, several observations can be observed from Table 9. First, the experimental group displayed a higher level of social skills than the control group did in the Combined, Kids, Male and Female Teens Samples. Second, the experimental group was less likely to abuse ketamine, sex, alcohol, smoking, and psychotropic substances than did the control group in the Male Kids Sample. Third, the experimental group perceived fewer benefits of abusing "ice" (Male Teens) than did the control group. Fourth, the experimental group displayed higher refusal skills than did the control group with reference to different drugs in the Combined, Kids, Male, Male Kids, Female Kids and Male Teens Samples.

Finally, the experimental group performed better than the control group on drug knowledge (Female Teens Sample) and sex knowledge (Male Sample). In terms of usage of drugs, there is evidence showing that the experimental group took less gateway drug than did the control group in the Female Sample, Male Kids Sample, and Female Kids Sample. With reference to the 52 significant findings in Table 9, 43 were positive findings. However, it has to be noted that although we can find a few interaction effects which were statistically significant in Tables 8 and 9 (pretest, posttest-1, and posttest-2), the effectiveness of the intervention was still not conclusive.

DISCUSSION

The findings reported above are basically positive and encouraging. Several aspects of the findings deserve attention. First, using different time points as reference points, there is evidence that the experimental group performed better than the control group in the domains of social skills, drug knowledge, sex knowledge, as well as drug-related and sex-related measures (including measures of attitudes, behavioral intention, refusal skills, and drug usage). These positive findings can be regarded as particularly encouraging because the experimental group was found to be worse than the control group in terms of drug-related measures at pretest. In view of the differences between the experimental group and control group at pretest, the positive changes in the experimental group can be regarded as substantial. Second, although some negative findings were observed with reference to the "pretest-posttest 1 dataset", such differences disappeared when the "pretest-posttest 1-posttest 2 dataset" were used as the bases of analyses. Third, the number of positive findings in different samples is much higher than the number of negative findings.

In brief, it was showed that the experimental group, after participating in the programs, was generally better than the control group in terms of social skills, knowledge of drugs, refusal skills, attitudes towards drugs, and the behavioral intention to avoid drug abuse. Although there were some negative findings, the number of positive findings was higher (i.e., about 63% of the 54 statistically significant findings summarized in Tables 4, 5, and 6). In view of the poorer performance of the experimental group at pretest, their positive changes at posttest can be regarded as an improvement that can contribute to the effects of the programs. Moreover, although some negative findings were observed in this pretest-posttest dataset, such differences disappeared when the second (six months later) posttest data were analyzed (see Tables 7, 8, and 9).

It should be noted that, first, the better performance of the experimental group relative to the control group varied across the samples (e.g., male kids performed better in the drug group, and male teens performed better in the non-drug group, refer to Tables 4 and 5). This finding suggests that the positive effects of the programs might be different for participants with different characteristics. Second, it was found that the Astro programs were more effective for non-drug participants - with the experimental group performing better in 75% of the 20 significant findings (compared with that of 53% of the 17 significant findings in the drug group). It suggests that this project could function well as drug prevention programs. On the other hand, there are some indicators for which the control group performed better than the experimental group. One possibility for such negative findings is that the subjects recruited in the experimental group were initially worse in terms of delinquency and drug-related behavior than those in the control group. These behaviors did not change in the program.

As far as the program evaluation is concerned and the present findings are encouraging, this study has two limitations. First, although a nonequivalent group design has been commonly used to evaluate drug prevention programs, its limitations should be recognized. Resources permitting, randomized controlled trials should be carried out to further evaluate the effectiveness of the Astro programs. Second, the present attempt is only able to evaluate the medium-term effects of the programs. It would be rewarding to examine the effectiveness of the programs over a longer period of time. Several studies have suggested the importance of conducting long-term evaluation studies to examine the effectiveness of structured drug prevention programs (9,22). In addition, since some of the popular drug prevention programs, such as the Drug Abuse Resistance Education (DARE) and Here's Looking at You 2000 (HLAY), have not yet demonstrated their effectiveness (23), long-term and vigorous evaluation studies are indispensable to provide useful information for evidence-based practice and policy formulation in the field of substance abuse prevention (21).

Despite these limitations, we were able to introduce the project and the model of preventive education to a number of social workers in Hong Kong and served well the purpose of enhancing the professional skills of practitioners. It is also encouraging that the participants in this study had changed in a positive direction after participating in the Astro programs. With reference to the comment made by Hanlon et al (24) that, in spite of the proliferation of drug abuse prevention strategies, there was little examination of conceptually based models under experimental and quasi-experimental conditions, our objective outcome evaluation study is an important addition to this area. The objective outcome evaluation findings constitute important additions to the limited literature on substance abuse prevention programs in a cross-cultural context. Moreover, there has so far been no evaluation research of drug prevention programs in Chinese communities (2), our study begins to eliminate this gap in the literature.

Obviously, the present study provides some initial evidence for a pioneer substance abuse prevention program in Hong Kong. One of the authors, Shek, has argued elsewhere thatit is important to take an evidence-based approach to evaluate the strategies to tackle adolescent substance abuse.Further discussion incorporating the ecological perspective, the concepts of riskand protective factors, preventions at the primary, secondary and tertiary levels, positive youth development, and holistic adolescent developmentare required, so that a more long-term and coordinated approach in tackling adolescent substance abuse can be carried out in future (25,26).

REFERENCES

[1] Shek DTL. The relation of parental qualities to psychological well-being, school adjustment, and problem behavior in Chinese adolescents with economic disadvantage. Am. J. Fam. Ther. 2002;30:215-30.

[2] Shek DTL, Lam MC, Tsoi KW. Evidence-based social work practice in Hong Kong. In:Thyer B, Kazi M, eds. International perspectives on evidence-based practice in social work. London: Venture Press, 2004:167-81.

[3] Glantz M. A developmental psychopathology model of drug abuse vulnerability. In: Glantz M, Pickens R, eds. Vulnerability to drug abuse. Washington, DC: Amercian Psychological Association, 1992:389-418.

[4] Hawkins JD, Catalano RF, Miller JY. Risk and protective factors for alcohol and other drug problems in adolescence and early adulthood: implications for substance abuse prevention. Psychol. Bull. 1992;112(1):64-105.

[5] McNeal JrR, Hansen WB. Developmental patterns associated with the onset of drug use: changes in postulated mediators during adolescence. J. Drug. Issues 1999;29(2):381-400.

[6] Stoil MJ, Hill G. Preventing substance abuse - Interventions that work. New York: Plenum, 1996.
[7] St Pierre TL, Kaltreider DL, Mark MM, Aikin KJ. Drug prevention in a community setting: alongitudinal study of the relative effectiveness of a three-year primary prevention program in Boys and Girls Clubs across the nation. Am. J. Commun. Psychol.1992;20:673-706.
[8] St Pierre TL, Kaltreider DL. Strategies for involving parents of high-risk youth in drug prevention: athree-year longitudinal study in Boys and Girls Clubs. J. Commun. Psychol. 1997;25(5):473-85.
[9] Lynam DR, Milich R, Zimmerman R, Novak SP, Logan TK, Martin C, et al. Project DARE: no effects at 10-year follow-up. J. Consult. Clin. Psychol. 1999;67:590-3.
[10] Rosenbaum DP, Hanson GS. Assessing the effects of school-based drug education: asix-year multilevel analysis of Project D.A.R.E. J. Res. Crime Delinq. 1998;35:381-412.
[11] Kaminski RA, Stromshak EA, Good RH, Goodman MR. Prevention of substance abuse with rural Head Start children and families: results of Project STAR. Psychol. Addict. Behav. 2002;16(Suppl 4):S11-26.
[12] Shek DTL, Ng HY, Lam CW, Lam OB, Yeung KC. A longitudinalevaluation study of a pioneering drug preventionprogram(Project Astro MIND) in Hong Kong. Hong Kong: Beat Drugs Fund and the Hong Kong Youth Institute, 2003.
[13] Creswell JW. Research designs: Qualitative, quantitative, and mixed method approaches. Thousand Oaks, CA: Sage, 2003.
[14] Patton MQ. Qualitative research and evaluation methods.Thousand Oaks: Sage, 2002.
[15] St Pierre TL, Kaltreider DL. SMART leaders handbook. University Park: Institute for Policy Research and Evaluation, The Pennsylvania State University, 1998.
[16] Rosenberg M. Conceiving the self. New York: Basic Books, 1979.
[17] Shek DTL. Family functioning and psychological well-being, school adjustment, and problem behavior in Chinese adolescents with and without economic disadvantage. J. Genet. Psychol.2002;16(3):497-502.
[18] St. Pierre TL, Kaltreider DL, Mark MM, Aikin KJ. Drug prevention in a community setting: alongitudinal study of the relative effectiveness of a three-year primary prevention program in Boys and Girls Clubs across the nation. Am. J. Commun. Psychol.1992;20:673-706.
[19] Tabachnick BG, Fidell LS. Using multivariate statistics. Boston: Allyn Bacon, 2001.
[20] Stevens JP. Applied multivariate statistics for the social sciences. Mahwah, NJ: Erlbaum, 2002.
[21] Gorman DM. The "science" of drug and alcohol prevention: the case of the randomized trial of the Life Skills Training program. Int. J. Drug Pol.2002;13:21-6.
[22] Rosenbaum DP, Hanson GS. Assessing the effects of school-based drug education: asix-year multilevel analysis of project D.A.R.E. J. Res. Crime Delinq.1998;35:381-412.
[23] Eisen M, Zellman GL, Massett HA, Murray DM. Evaluating the Lions-Quest "Skills for Adolescence" drug education program: first-year behavior outcomes. Addict. Behav. 2002;27:619-32.

[24] Hanlon TE, Bateman RW, Simon BD, O'Grady KE, Carswell SB. An early community-based intervention for the prevention and substance abuse and other delinquent behavior. J. Youth Adolesc. 2002;31:459-71.
[25] Shek DTL. Tackling adolescent substance abuse in Hong Kong: where we should and should not go. ScientificWorld Journal2007;7:2021-30.
[26] Shek DTL. School drug testing: a critical review of the literature. ScientificWorld Journal 2010;10:356-65.

In: Drug Abuse in Hong Kong
Editors: D Shek, R Sun and J Merrick

ISBN: 978-1-61324-491-3
©2012 Nova Science Publishers, Inc.

Chapter 5

PERSPECTIVE AND SUBJECTIVE OUTCOME OF THE PROGRAM FROM THE PARTICIPANTS

Daniel TL Shek[1,a,b,c,d,e] and Chiu-Wan Lam[a]

[a]Department of Applied Social Sciences,
The Hong Kong Polytechnic University, Hong Kong, PRC
[b]Public Policy Research Institute,
The Hong Kong Polytechnic University, Hong Kong, PRC
[c]East China Normal University, Shanghai, PRC
[d]Kiang Wu Nursing College of Macau, Macau, PRC
[e]Division of Adolescent Medicine, Department of Pediatrics,
Kentucky Children's Hospital, University of Kentucky,
College of Medicine, Lexington, Kentucky, US

ABSTRACT

A total of 106 and 175 participants participated in the Astro Kids and Astro Teens Programs of Project Astro MIND in Hong Kong, respectively. After completion of the programs, participants were invited to respond to a subjective outcome evaluation form to assess their views of the program in terms of information giving, arrangement of the program, performance of the

---

[1]Correspondence: Professor Daniel TL Shek, PhD, FHKPS, BBS, JP, Chair Professor, Department of Applied Social Sciences, The Hong Kong Polytechnic University, Hunghom, Hong Kong. E-mail: daniel.shek@polyu.edu.hk.

workers, and perceived effectiveness. Results showed that most of the participants had positive perceptions of different aspects of the programs and the instructors. There were high proportions of the participants who viewed that the program had helped them acquire healthier attitude towards refusing drugs, enhance their drug knowledge and improve drug refusal skills, drug refusal behavior and social skills. The subjective outcome evaluation findings based on the perspective of the participants provide support for the effectiveness of the Astro Program in Hong Kong.

INTRODUCTION

Probably because of the influence of popular culture and youth sub-culture as well as disintegration of families, substance abuse among young people has become an acute global problem. As Hong Kong is an international city where information flow (including those related to psychotropic drugs) is very quick, adolescent substance abuse is also a grave concern for Hong Kong (1). An examination of the substance abuse figures in the past twenty years showed that there were three peaks in the substance abusers figures reported to the Central Registry of Drug Abuse (CRDA) maintained by the Narcotics Division of the Government of the Hong Kong Special Administrative Region. The first peak was in mid-1990s which was mainly related to easy access to tranquilizers which were not tightly controlled by legislations. The second peak was in early 2000s which was closely related to the rave party culture. The third peak was in 2008-09 which was mainly related to abuse of ketamine in schools. In fact, these peaks mirrored the global trend of abusing non-opiate psychotropic substances and the growing belief among young people that psychotropic substance abuse is non-addictive and it is a valid choice of life. The number of young people abusing psychotropic substances has increased in the past decade. In the recent school survey conducted by the Narcotics Division, it was found that drug abuse was more prevalent than those reported in previous studies, although the prevalence rates were still not as high as those in Western countries.

With the intensification of adolescent substance abuse in Hong Kong, there is a demand for adolescent substance abuse prevention programs (2, 3). Although many organizations in Hong Kong provide drug prevention programs for young people, such programs often lack vigorous evaluation. To help high-risk adolescents to stay away from drugs, the Beat Drugs Fund of the Government of the Hong Kong Special Administrative Region and Wofoo Foundation supported a project entitled "Project Astro" undertaken by researchers of The University of Hong Kong and The Chinese University of Hong Kong (4, 5). In this paper, the

Table 1. Design and content of the Astro Program

Program	Astro Kids	Astro Teens	Astro Leaders	Astro Club
Age range	10-13	13-16	Graduates of Astro Teens	Graduates of Astro programs
No. of sessions	10	12	"3 + 1" community involvement project	---
Content	Stress and coping, family relationship, smoking, drug education, puberty, friendship, refusal skills, self-understanding, pressure from media.	Stress and coping, decision-making, gateway drugs, drug education, teenage sex, self-image, refusal skills, peer pressure, life planning.	Self-image, life planning, community involvement project.	Healthy activities and building up of support network among members.

development of a pioneering drug prevention program in Hong Kong (Project Astro MIND) is described and evaluation findings pertinent to the effectiveness of the related programs are presented. Project Astro MIND comprises three sequential and developmentally appropriate programs (Astro Kids, Astro Teens, and Astro Leaders) designed for children and adolescents, with topics on drug, sex, adolescent development, and life skills with reference to risk and protective factors in adolescent substance abuse are included in the group sessions. For the graduates of the programs, they can join programs on leaders and with the involvement of the family members. The design of the program can be seen in Table 1.

To understand the effectiveness of the project, there are at least four evaluation questions that should be asked: a) Are there any positive changes in the program participants (i.e., objective outcome evaluation)? b) Are the program participants and workers satisfied with the program (i.e., subjective outcome evaluation)? c) What happens during the program implementation process (i.e., process evaluation)? d) What are the subjective experiences of the program participants and the workers (i.e., qualitative evaluation)? Definitely, the inclusion of different evaluation mechanisms may help to triangulate the findings collected.

As far as objective outcome evaluation is concerned, a quasi-experimental longitudinal design was employed to evaluate the effectiveness of the project. For participants in the experimental groups (139 Astro Kids and 217 Astro Teens participants) and the control groups (213 Astro Kids and 201 Astro Teens controls), they were required to respond to objective outcome measures, including measures of social skills, attitude towards drugs, refusal skills towards drugs, usage of drugs, behavioral intention, drug and sex knowledge, stress and psychological well-being at pretest and different posttests. Analyses of covariance controlling for pretest differences showed that Astro Kids and Astro Teens programs were effective in increasing the social skills, refusal skills, drug knowledge and sex knowledge of the participants. Compared with control participants, program participants also had less favorable attitudes towards taking drugs at posttest (4, 5).

Besides objective outcome evaluation, subjective outcome evaluation is commonly used to examine subjective experiences of the program participants. In human services, the importance of involving the service users or program participants in evaluation is advocated, and thus subjective outcome evaluation becomes popularly used to capture the viewpoints of the participants. In regard of this, client satisfaction surveys are commonly used as a feedback for transforming services to meet the users' needs for planning and administration purposes, or simply used as an indicator of program effectiveness from the participants' perspective for research purpose. Although there are many criticisms of this approach, the client satisfaction approach is widely used in different service settings (6, 7). As pointed out by Royse (8), "despite the generally positive bias and the problems associated with collecting representative samples of clients, there is much to recommend client satisfaction studies as one means of evaluating a program. Because professionals do not experience the agency in the same way as the clients, it is important to ask clients to share their experiences" (p.264-265).

Subjective outcome evaluation is a commonly used strategy to evaluate programs in the context of human services and it has been used by different professionals in different fields, such as education, social work, psychology, medicine, and allied health professions. The commonly used approach is to develop closed-ended rating scale items to quantify client satisfaction. For example, standardized rating scales, such as the Medical Interview Satisfaction Scale, Consumer Satisfaction Questionnaire, and Client Satisfaction Questionnaire were developed to gauge client satisfaction and perceived helpfulness of the program (9).

There are findings suggesting that the linkage between objective outcome and subjective outcome evaluation findings is strong, therefore underscoring the utility of subjective outcome evaluation findings. Based on the responses of 546 students participated in a positive youth development program in Hong Kong, Shek et al. (10) showed that subjective outcome evaluation measures were significantly related to objective measures of positive youth development. In another study, Shek (11) examined the convergence between subjective outcome evaluation measures and objective outcome evaluation measures in 3,298 Chinese secondary school students in Hong Kong. Results showed that the subjective outcome measures were significantly correlated with posttest scores and difference scores based on measures of objective outcome indicators and they also predicted changes in CPYDS scores across time. Shek (11) concluded that the present findings demystify the common belief that findings based on the client satisfaction approach are unrelated to objective outcome evaluation findings.

Adopting the principle of triangulation, different types of data based on different evaluation strategies were utilized in the Project Astro. In the present study, subjective outcome evaluation data based on the participants joining the Astro Kids and Astro Teens programs were reported. It was expected that through subjective outcome evaluation findings, the views of the program through the perspective of the program participants were explored.

OUR PROJECT

In this project, subjective outcome indicators were used to gauge the perceived benefits and levels of satisfaction of the program participants regarding the different aspects of the program. After completion of the program, the group members were invited to respond to global structured questionnaires measuring their perceptions of the benefits of and satisfaction with the program.

For both Astro Kids and Astro Teens programs, the respondents were asked to evaluate the program after each session and after the completion of the training. For the Global Subjective Outcomes Evaluation Form for Astro Kids program, the participants were asked to indicate their satisfaction with and perception of the qualities of the program (Question 1) as well as the evaluation of helpfulness of the program (Question 2). Besides, the respondents were asked to indicate whether the program could help them to distance themselves from smoking (Question 6), other drugs (Question 7), and sexual behavior (Question 8). They were also asked to respond to three open-ended questions, including their perceptions of the most important things they have learned (Question 3), things that should be improved (Question 4), and whether the participant would recommend the program to their friends (Question 5). The Global Subjective Outcomes Evaluation Form for the Astro Teens program was basically the same with some minor modifications. A total of 106 and 175 questionnaires were collected from the participants joining the Astro Kids and Astro Teens programs, respectively.

WHAT THE PARTICIPANTS TOLD US

Subjective outcomes based on participants of the Astro Kids Program (N=106)

The findings on the participants' evaluation of the details of the program are shown in Table 2 to Table 7. As shown in Table 2, most of the participants were satisfied with the provision of information (89% were satisfied or very satisfied), arrangements of the day camp (71% were satisfied or very satisfied), provision of materials (90% were satisfied or very satisfied), worker's performance (85% were satisfied or very satisfied), refreshments (81% were satisfied or very satisfied), arrangement of group activities (86% were satisfied or very satisfied), and other activities (83% were satisfied or very satisfied). Furthermore, most of them were of the view that qualities of the different aspects of the program were good or very good with respect to the provision of information (85%), arrangements of the day camp (72%), provision of materials (82%), worker's performance (83%), refreshments (81%), arrangement of group activities (79%), and arrangement of other activities (84%).

Generally speaking, most of the participants felt that the program was either helpful or very helpful for adolescents in the areas of drug refusal attitudes (86%), improvement of drug refusal skills (88%), drug refusal behavior (89%), increase in social skills (87%), and increase of drug knowledge (90%). The findings can be seen in Table 3.

Similarly, most of the participants held the views that the program could help group members to distance them from smoking (88% of the responses were "Helpful" or "Very Helpful"), usage of other drugs (93% of the responses were "Helpful" or "Very Helpful") as well as early sex (89% of the responses were "Helpful" or "Very Helpful"). The related findings are presented in Table 7.

The responses to the three open-ended questions can be seen in Table 4 to Table 6. To enhance the reliability of the coding, a certain proportion of the responses to each question were randomly selected for inter-rater reliability checking. The findings suggest that the coding systems adopted were reliable.

Table 2. Degree of satisfaction with and perceived qualities of the program among participants of the Astro Kids program (N=106)

	Level of Satisfaction					Qualities of the Program				
	Very Dissatisfied	Dissatisfied	Satisfied	Very Satisfied	Missing value	Very Poor	Poor	Good	Very Good	Missing Value
Information giving	5%	5%	50%	39%	1%	5%	5%	47%	38%	5%
Arrangement of day camp activities	5%	6%	38%	33%	18%	3%	7%	39%	33%	18%
Resources giving	3%	6%	43%	47%	1%	1%	13%	41%	41%	4%
Performance of workers	6%	7%	41%	44%	2%	6%	7%	43%	40%	4%
Refreshments	6%	7%	35%	46%	6%	3%	7%	36%	45%	9%
Arrangement of the program (e.g., place, activities, time, etc.)	4%	7%	33%	53%	3%	3%	13%	30%	49%	5%
Other activities	7%	3%	42%	41%	7%	2%	5%	42%	42%	9%

Table 3. Perceived degree of helpfulness of the Astro Kids program by the participants

	Degree of Helpfulness			
	Not At All Helpful	Slightly Helpful	Helpful	Very Helpful
Attitude towards refusing drugs	7%	7%	41%	45%
Improvement of refusal skills towards drugs	6%	6%	40%	48%
Behavior on refusing drugs	4%	7%	37%	52%
Improvement of social skills	4%	9%	50%	37%
Enhancement of drug knowledge	3%	7%	37%	53%

Table 4. Participants' perceptions of the most important things that they had learned from the Astro Kids program

No.	Items	Responses(N)	Percentage
1	Not to take drugs	22	16%
2	Refusal skills	13	9%

Table 4. (Continued)

No.	Items	Responses(N)	Percentage
3	Harmful effect of smoking	13	9%
4	Drug knowledge	11	8%
5	Harmful effect of abusing drugs	11	8%
6	Learned much knowledge	7	5%
7	Sex knowledge	6	4%
8	Communication with others	6	4%
9	Self understanding	5	4%
10	Friendship	3	2%
11	Learning how to communicate with family members	3	2%
12	Peer pressure affecting personal development	3	2%
13	Coping with stress	2	2%
14	Differentiating right and wrong	2	2%
15	Expressing personal views	1	1%
16	No comments	31	22%
Total		139	100%

Remarks: Out of 35 randomly selected responses, the first rater and second rater agreed on 30 responses over the classification (inter-rater reliability= 85.71%).

Table 5. Comments and suggestions from members on how the Astro Kids program could be improved

No.	Items	Responses (N)	Percentage
1	More activities	5	5%
2	Longer period of time	4	4%
3	Increase the number of group members	2	2%
4	Control the noise among group members	2	2%
5	Improving personal attitude	2	2%
6	More prize-giving	2	2%
7	Improving the performance of workers	1	1%
8	Improving the relationship among group members	1	1%
9	More interaction among group members	1	1%
10	Larger places for group work activities	1	1%
11	More refreshments	1	1%
12	Improving social skills	1	1%
13	No comments	83	77%
Total		106	100%

Remarks: Out of 20 randomly selected responses, the first rater and second rater agreed on 18 responses over the classification (inter-rater reliability= 90%).

Table 6. Degree of willingness of the members to recommend the Astro Kids program to other people

No.	Items	Responses (N)	Percentage
1	Yes	72	68%
2	No	16	15%
3	Possibly	1	1%
4	No comments	17	16%
Total		106	100%

Remarks: Out of 20 randomly selected responses, the first rater and second rater agreed on 20 responses over the classification (inter-rater reliability= 100%).

Table 7. Perceptions of the degree of helpfulness of the Astro Kids program amongst the participants

	Degree of Helpfulness				
	Not At All Helpful	Slightly Helpful	Helpful	Very Helpful	Missing Value
Do you think "Astro Kids" can help you to stay away from smoking?	3%	7%	31%	57%	2%
Do you think "Astro Kids" can help you to stay away from drugs (e.g., Cannabis, Heroin, Ketamine, MDMA, "Ice")?	1%	5%	25%	68%	1%
Do you think "Astro Kids" can help you to prevent early sex?	3%	7%	30%	59%	1%

Subjective outcomes based on participants of the Astro Teens Program (N=175)

The findings on the participants' evaluation of the details of the program are shown in Table 8 to Table 13. From Table 8, results showed that most of the participants were satisfied with the provision of information (92% were satisfied or very satisfied), arrangements of the day camp (74% were satisfied or very satisfied), provision of materials (87% were satisfied or very satisfied), worker's performance (92% were satisfied or very satisfied), refreshments (74% were satisfied or very satisfied), arrangement of group activities (78% were satisfied or very satisfied), and other activities (82% were satisfied or very satisfied). Furthermore, most of them were of the view that qualities of different aspects of the program were good or very good with respect to the provision of information (87%), arrangements of the day camp (72%), provision of materials (87%), worker's performance (88%), refreshments (73%), and arrangement of group activities (77%).

Table 8. Degree of satisfaction with and perceived qualities of the program among participants of the Astro Teens program (N=175)

	Level of Satisfaction					Perceived Qualities			
	Very Dis-satisfied	Dis-satisfied	Satisfied	Very Satisfied	Missing value	Very Poor	Poor	Good	Very Good	Missing Value
Information giving	3%	4%	69%	23%	1%	1%	6%	69%	18%	6%
Arrangement of day camp activities	3%	14%	51%	23%	9%	0%	13%	49%	23%	15%
Resources giving	3%	9%	65%	22%	1%	1%	8%	65%	22%	4%
Performance of workers	1%	5%	57%	35%	2%	1%	5%	56%	32%	6%
Refreshments	4%	14%	47%	27%	8%	4%	10%	51%	22%	13%
Arrangement of the program (e.g., place, activities, time, etc.)	2%	18%	56%	22%	2%	1%	17%	56%	21%	5%
Other activities	1%	9%	57%	25%	8%	1%	10%	56%	22%	11%

Table 9. Perceived degree of helpfulness of the Astro Teens program by the participants

	Degree of Helpfulness				
	Not At All Helpful	Slightly Helpful	Helpful	Very Helpful	Missing value
Attitude towards refusing drugs	3%	11%	60%	26%	0%
Improvement of refusal skills towards drugs	2%	13%	53%	31%	1%
Behavior on refusing drugs	3%	15%	49%	32%	1%
Improvement of social skills	3%	14%	52%	31%	0%
Enhancement of drug knowledge	2%	9%	47%	42%	0%

Generally speaking, most of the participants felt that the program was either helpful or very helpful for adolescents in the areas of drug refusal attitudes (86%), improvement of drug refusal skills (84%), drug refusal behavior (81%), increase in social skills (83%), and increase of drug knowledge (89%). The results can be seen in Table 9. Similarly, most of the participants held the views that the program could help group members to distance them from smoking (74% of the responses were "Helpful" or "Very Helpful"), drinking (73% of the responses were "Helpful" or "Very Helpful"), usage of other drugs (86% of the responses were "Helpful" or "Very Helpful") and early sex (78% of the responses were "Helpful" or "Very Helpful"). The related findings are presented in Table 10.

Table 10. Perceptions of the degree of helpfulness of the Astro Teens program among the participants

	Level of Helpfulness				
	Not At All Helpful	Slightly Helpful	Helpful	Very Helpful	Missing Value
Do you think "Astro Teens" can help you to stay away from smoking?	10%	15%	46%	28%	1%
Do you think "Astro Teens" program can help you to stay away from alcohol?	10%	16%	47%	26%	1%
Do you think "Astro Teens" can help you to stay away from drugs (e.g., Cannabis, Heroin, Ketamine, MDMA, "Ice")?	5%	8%	42%	44%	1%
Do you think "Astro Teens" can help you to prevent early sex?	11%	10%	42%	36%	1%

The responses to the three open-ended questions can be seen in Table 11 to Table 13. To enhance the reliability of the coding, a certain proportion of the responses to each question were randomly selected for inter-rater reliability checking. The findings suggest that the coding systems adopted were reliable.

Table 11. Participants' perceptions of the most important things that they had learned from the Astro Teens program

No.	Items	Responses (N)	Percentage
1	Drug knowledge	23	11%
2	Harmful effect of abusing drugs	19	9%

Table 11. (Continued)

No.	Items	Responses N)	Percentage
3	Not to take drugs	19	9%
4	Team spirit and co-operation	17	8%
5	Sex knowledge	16	7%
6	Refusal skills	13	6%
7	Understanding other group members	6	3%
8	Improving social skills	6	3%
9	Self understanding	6	3%
10	Learning to get along with others	6	3%
11	Respecting other people	4	2%
12	Harmful effect of smoking	4	2%
13	Emotional control	3	1%
14	Taking care of others	2	1%
15	Learning different knowledge	2	1%
16	Choosing friends	2	1%
17	Procedure and methods on decision-making	1	0%
18	Setting up goal	1	0%
19	Expressing personal view	1	0%
20	Improving family relationship	1	0%
21	Releasing stress	1	0%
22	No comments	66	30%
Total		219	100%

Remarks: Out of 45 randomly selected responses, the first rater and second rater agreed on 40 responses over the classification (inter-rater reliability= 88.89%).

Table 12. Comments and suggestions from members for improving Astro Teens program

No.	Items	Responses (N)	Percentage
1	More refreshments	18	9%
2	More exciting activities	17	9%
3	More outdoor activities such as over-night camp	17	9%
4	Better time management	16	7%
5	More group sessions	4	2%
6	Improving the arrangement for the program venue	3	2%
7	More interaction among group members	2	1%
8	Increasing the number of group members	2	1%
9	Reducing the number of questionnaires	2	1%
10	Group members have the right to choose	1	1%
11	More prize-giving	1	1%
12	Arranging more voluntary services	1	1%
13	No comments	110	56%
Total		194	100%

Remarks: Out of 40 randomly selected responses, the first rater and second rater agreed on 34 responses over the classification (inter-rater reliability= 85%).

Table 13. Degree of willingness of the members to recommend the Astro Teens program to other people

No.	Items	Responses (N)	Percentage
1	Yes	107	61%
2	No	21	12%
3	Possibly	4	2%
4	No comments	43	25%
	Total	175	100%

Remarks: Out of 35 randomly selected responses, the first rater and second rater agreed on 35 responses over the classification (inter-rater reliability= 100%).

DISCUSSION

Subjective outcome evaluation or client satisfaction survey is commonly used to assess the perceived benefits of a program and the degree of satisfaction that the participants have regarding different aspects of the program. The use of subjective outcome indicators or the client satisfaction approach in evaluation has a long history in human services in different cultures. Although there are arguments against the use of subjective outcome assessment, there is evidence showing that subjective outcome measures were correlated with objective outcome measures (10, 11).

The findings based on the subjective outcome evaluation strategy or client satisfaction survey showed that a high proportion of the respondents had positive perceptions of the program and the worker. Most importantly, most of the respondents regarded the program as helpful to them. In short, the subjective outcome evaluation findings generally showed that the program participants had positive perception of the program as well as the workers who implemented the program.

There are three strengths of this study. First, the subjective outcome evaluation findings are based on two samples comprising of kids and teenagers. The inclusion of these two samples can help us further understand the perceived effectiveness of the programs in children and adolescents. Second, different aspects of subjective outcome, including views on the program, worker, perceived effectiveness, and overall satisfaction were covered in the study. Third, the present study demonstrates the importance of assessing reliability in qualitative data analyses. In fact, there are few attempts examining reliability in subjective outcome evaluation finings. This study is the first published scientific study in a drug prevention program in the Chinese culture.

Of course, several limitations of the present study should be highlighted (12-16). First, although the sample of participants in the study was not small, there is a need to replicate the findings in different populations. Second, while the present findings are interpreted in terms of the positive program effects and experiences of the program participants, it should be noted that there are several alternative explanations. The first alternative explanation is that the participants were afraid that they might disappoint the workers, therefore responding in the favorable direction. Actually, this alternative explanation can be partially dismissed because the participants responded in an anonymous manner. The second alternative explanation is that the students consciously acted in a "nice" manner to help the workers to illustrate positive program effect. However, this alternative explanation could be partially dismissed because negative ratings were recorded and the participants responded in an anonymous manner. The third alternative explanation is that the high proportion of positive responses observed was in fact random responses. However, this alternative explanation can also be dismissed because reliability analyses showed that the responses were coherent in nature. Despite these limitations, the present findings suggest that the Astro Kids and Astro Teens and its implementation were perceived in a positive manner by the program participants and they perceived the program to be beneficial to their own development. These positive findings are important because there are few effective adolescent drug prevention programs in different Chinese communities.

REFERENCES

[1] Shek DTL. Tackling adolescent substance abuse in Hong Kong: where we should and should not go. ScientificWorld Journal 2007;7:2021-30.
[2] Shek DTL. International conferenceon tackling drug abuse: Conference proceedings. Hong Kong: Narcotics Division, Security Bureau, Government of Hong Kong Special Administrative Region, 2006.
[3] Shek DTL. School drug testing: a critical review of the literature. Scientific World Journal 2010;10:356-65.
[4] Lam CW, Shek DTL, Ng HY, Yeung KC, Lam DOB. An innovation in drug prevention programs for adolescents: the Hong Kong Astro Project. Int. J. Adolesc. Med. Health 2005;17(4):343-53.
[5] Shek DTL, Ng HY, Lam CW, Lam OB, Yeung KC. A longitudinal evaluation study of a pioneering drug preventionprogram (Project Astro MIND) in Hong Kong. Hong Kong: Beat Drugs Fund and the Hong Kong Youth Institute, 2003.
[6] Ginsberg LH. Social work evaluation. Boston, MA: Allyn Bacon, 2001.
[7] Weinbach RW. Evaluating social work services and programs. Boston, MA: Allyn Bacon, 2005.

[8] Royse D. Research methods in social work. Pacific Grove, CA: Brooks/Cole, 2004.
[9] Shek DTL, Sun RCF. Subjective outcome evaluation based on secondary data analyses: the Project P.A.T.H.S. in Hong Kong. Scientific World Journal 2010;10:224-37.
[10] Shek DTL, Lee TY, Siu AMH, Ma HK. Convergence of subjective outcome and objective outcome evaluation findings: insights based on the Project P.A.T.H.S. .Scientific World Journal 2007;7:258-67.
[11] Shek DTL. Subjective outcome and objective outcome evaluation findings: insights from a Chinese context. Res. Soc. Work Pract. 2010;20(3):293-301.
[12] Ma HK, Shek DTL. Subjective outcome evaluation of a positive youth development program in Hong Kong: profiles and correlates. Scientific World Journal 2010;10:192-200.
[13] Shek DTL, Ma CMS. Subjective outcome evaluation findings: factors related to the perceived effectiveness of the Tier 2 Program of the Project P.A.T.H.S..Scientific World Journal 2010;10:250-60.
[14] Shek DTL, Yu L. Subjective outcome evaluation of the Project P.A.T.H.S.: descriptive profiles and correlates. Scientific World Journal 2010;10:211-23.
[15] Shek DTL. Quantitative evaluation of the training program of the Project P.A.T.H.S. in Hong Kong. Int. J. Adolesc. Med. Health 2010;22(3):425-35.
[16] Shek DTL, Chak YYL. Design of training programs for a positive youth development program: Project P.A.T.H.S. in Hong Kong. Int. J. Adolesc. Med. Health 2010; 22 (3): 345-67.

In: Drug Abuse in Hong Kong
Editors: D Shek, R Sun and J Merrick
ISBN: 978-1-61324-491-3
©2012 Nova Science Publishers, Inc.

Chapter 6

PERSPECTIVE OF THE SOCIAL WORKERS IN OUTCOME EVALUATION OF A DRUG PREVENTION PROGRAM IN HONG KONG

Chiu-Wan Lam[1,a] *and Daniel TL Shek*[a,b,c,d,e]
[a]Department of Applied Social Sciences,
The Hong Kong Polytechnic University, Hong Kong, PRC
[b]Public Policy Research Institute,
The Hong Kong Polytechnic University, Hong Kong, PRC
[c]East China Normal University, Shanghai, PRC
[d]Kiang Wu Nursing College of Macau, Macau, PRC
[e]Division of Adolescent Medicine, Department of Pediatrics,
Kentucky Children's Hospital, University of Kentucky,
College of Medicine, Lexington, Kentucky, US

ABSTRACT

Subjective outcome evaluation was carried out for workers implementing the Astro Kids and Astro Teens designed for high-risk youth in Hong Kong. Each social worker was invited to fill out a self-administered feedback form after each session. In addition, each respondent was asked to

---

[1] Correspondence: Chiu-Wan Lam, PhD, Department of Applied Social Sciences, The Hong Kong Polytechnic University, Hunghom, Hong Kong. E-mail: sscwlam@polyu.edu.hk.

complete a Global Subjective Outcome Evaluation Form after the completion of the training program. The subjective outcome evaluation data regarding the global evaluation of the Astro Teens and Astro Kids programs clearly indicate that most of the social workers were satisfied with the programs. They also perceived many positive features of the programs and felt that they were helpful in terms of knowledge acquisition, healthy attitude formation, and building resistance against substance abuse.

INTRODUCTION

It can be envisaged that with a change in perspective in how addiction is to be seen, from the medical perspective to the cognitive, the role of social work can potentially range from counselling in drug treatment and rehabilitation centers, to preventive and educational programs in the community. For the drug addicts must be seen as having impaired capacity to cope with life circumstances, such that they will need a process of rehabilitation involving the re-building of a whole different life style (1). This is an area where the social work profession can contribute significantly towards the restoration of impaired capacity, provision of individual and social resources to former abusers for re-integrating into society. In the area of drug prevention for the high-risk groups, if the importance of their family members is taken into account and they need to be involved to help them for the cultivation of protective factors, the importance of social workers in this area will probably be found scattered across family and child service.

In view of the increasing involvement of young people in drugs, social workers will all be essential to help prevent them from drug addiction. Social workers involved in schools and youth work will have an important role to play in alerting society to conditions that make for potential drug abuse, as there are studies indicating that leaving school at an early age and involvement in criminal activities are related to drug use. Necessary steps to address these circumstances, for example, through involvement in preventive and educational programs by social workers, have been acknowledged. There is also a continuous need to see preventive education in the context of young people's life-style, not as related only to drug abuse. Also in evaluating educational programs in schools in the United States, it was long since discovered, and has continued to be so, that direct teaching about drugs and the problem of abuse was ineffective (2). Instead, those that stressed both environmental and individual factors, general life skills and value clarification were successful in reducing the number of teenagers from entering into drug (3, 4).

With the above-said concerns in mind and conscious of the need to develop a drug prevention program that is evidence-based, systematic, and indigenous to Chinese culture, the Project Astro was designed by the authors and their research team in Hong Kong (5). We introduced the project, its programs, and the model of preventive education to a number of children and youth service centers in Hong Kong. It was found that social workers, with their broad-based training which enabled them to engage in a diverse set of interventive tasks, were basically well prepared for drug prevention work. Their background training in developmental models and social skills training also equipped them for such tasks without difficulty. On the other hand, with reference to the comment made by Shek et al. (5) that, in spite of the proliferation of drug abuse prevention strategies, evaluation research of drug prevention programs in Chinese communities was scarce. This evaluation research of a drug prevention program aims at constituting an important addition to this area, and we will focus on the subjective evaluation outcomes of the social workers who have implemented the Astro programs.

OUR PROJECT

Subjective outcome evaluations or client satisfaction surveys are commonly used to assess the perceived benefits of the program and the degree of satisfaction with it. The use of subjective outcome indicators or the user satisfaction approach in evaluation has a long history in human services in different cultures (6-9). Although there are arguments against the use of subjective outcome assessment (10), evidence exists showing the correlation between subjective outcome measures and objective outcome measures (11-17). In this project, subjective outcome indicators were used to gauge the perceived benefits and levels of satisfaction of social workers. At the completion of the program, social workers were invited to respond to global structured questionnaires measuring their responses to the program.

For both the Astro Kids and Astro Teens programs, the respondents were asked to evaluate the program after each session and the completion of the training. There were two similar evaluation forms for the social workers, one for the Astro Kids program and another for the Astro Teens program. In the Global Subjective Outcomes Evaluation Form for the Astro Kids program, social workers were asked to indicate their satisfaction with the components of the program, including information giving (Question 1), arrangement of daycamp (Question 2), resources giving (Question 3), arrangement of refreshments (Question 5), and program activities (Question 6). The respondents were also asked whether they think the overall performance of the social work team of the programs was satisfactory (Question 4). The social workers were also asked to respond to three open-ended questions about their perceptions of the most important things that participants of the program had learned (Question A), things that should be improved (Question B), and whether the participant would recommend the program to other people (Question C). The Global Subjective Outcomes Evaluation Form for the Astro Teens program was similar, with some minor modifications.

THE EVALUATION BY THE SOCIAL WORKERS

The findings on the social workers' evaluation (N=13) of the program details are shown in Tables 1 and 2. As Table1 shows, most were satisfied with the provision of information (100% were satisfied or very satisfied), arrangements of the day camp (39% were satisfied and 46% had no opinion), provision of materials (100% were satisfied or very satisfied), workers' performance (92% were satisfied), refreshments (100% were satisfied or very satisfied), arrangement of the program (100% were satisfied), and arrangement of other activities (69% were satisfied). With reference to the qualities of the program, most respondents felt the program was good or very good with respect to the provision of information (92%), arrangements of the day camp (39% responded "Good" and 46% had no opinion), provision of materials (100%), workers' performance (92%), refreshments (100%), arrangement of the program (92%), and arrangement of other activities (69%). Overall speaking, the qualities of the program activities were well received by most of the social workers.

Most of the workers felt that the program was either helpful or very helpful for adolescents in the areas of drug refusal attitudes (85%), improvement of drug refusal skills (85%), drug refusal behavior (62%), improvement of social skills (85%), and increase of drug knowledge (92%). Similarly, most of the workers believed that the program could help group members refrain from smoking (84% of the responses were "Helpful" or "Very Helpful"), using other drugs (92% of the responses were "Helpful" or "Very Helpful"), and engaging in early sex (77% of the responses were "Helpful" or "Very Helpful"). The findings are displayed in Table 2.

Table 1. Degree of satisfaction with and perceived qualities of the program amongst workers of the Astro Kids program (N=13)

	Level of Satisfaction					Perceived Qualities			
	Very Dissatisfied	Dissatisfied	Satisfied	Very Satisfied	Missing value	Very Poor	Poor	Good	Very Good	Missing Value
Information giving	0%	0%	85%	15%	0%	0%	8%	77%	15%	0%
Arrangement of day camp activities	0%	15%	39%	0%	46%	0%	15%	39%	0%	46%
Resources giving	0%	0%	69%	31%	0%	0%	0%	92%	8%	0%
Performance of workers	0%	8%	92%	0%	0%	0%	8%	92%	0%	0%
Refreshments	0%	0%	92%	8%	0%	0%	0%	92%	8%	0%
Arrangement of the program (e.g., place, activities, time, etc.)	0%	0%	100%	0%	0%	0%	0%	92%	0%	8%
Other activities	0%	0%	69%	0%	31%	0%	0%	69%	0%	31%

Table 2. Perceived degree of helpfulness of the Astro Kids program by the workers (N=13)

	Degree of Helpfulness			
	Not At All Helpful	Slightly Helpful	Helpful	Very Helpful
Attitude toward refusing drugs	0%	15%	54%	31%
Improvement of refusal skills towards drugs	0%	15%	39%	46%
Behavior on refusing drugs	0%	38%	54%	8%
Improvement of social skills	0%	15%	62%	23%
Enhancement of drug knowledge	0%	8%	69%	23%
Do you think "Astro Kids" program can help members to stay away from smoking?	8%	8%	46%	38%
Do you think "Astro Kids" program can help members to stay away from drugs (e.g., Cannabis, Heroin, Ketamine, MDMA, "Ice") ?	0%	8%	61%	31%
Do you think "Astro Kids" can help members to prevent early sex?	8%	15%	62%	15%

Table 3. The responses of social workers of Astro Kids program to the open-ended questions

No.		Responses (N)	%
a. Workers' perceptions of the most important things that participants of the Astro Kids program had learned from the program			
1	Drug knowledge	6	27%
2	Refusal skills	4	18%
3	Awareness of the harmful effect of gateway drugs	2	9%
4	Interaction with others	2	9%
5	Sex knowledge	2	9%
6	Respecting other people	1	4%
7	Listen to others	1	4%
8	Understanding of how people and things affect personal development	1	4%
9	Coping with peer pressure	1	4%
10	Following group norms	1	4%
11	Emotional control	1	4%
12	No comments	1	4%
Total		23	100%
b. Workers' suggestions on how the Astro Kids program can be improved			
1	Reduction of activities that require writing	3	17%
2	Modify activities in the manuals	2	12%
3	More group sessions	1	6%
4	Reduction of abstract concepts and focusing more on discussion and sharing sessions	1	6%
5	Strengthening positive reinforcement from peers	1	6%
6	Revising the content of the session on sex because it is difficult to understand	1	6%
7	Reduction of activities and topics in the manuals	1	6%
8	Members joining the group on a voluntary bases	1	6%
9	Replacing "Astro Film" activities in each session by direct conversation between facilitators and group members	1	6%
10	Recruitment of both "normal" youth and youth with deviant behavior at the same time	1	6%
11	Group activities suiting the characteristics of target groups	1	6%
12	No comments	3	17%
Total		17	100%
c. Workers' willingness to recommend the Astro Kids program to other people			
1	Yes	9	70%
2	No	2	15%
3	No comments	2	15%
Total		13	100%

Remarks:
a. Out of 10 randomly selected responses, the first rater and second rater agreed on 8 responses over the classification (inter-rater reliability= 80%).
b. Out of 8 randomly selected responses, the first rater and second rater agreed on 6 responses over the classification (inter-rater reliability= 75%).
c. Out of 13 randomly selected responses, the first rater and second rater agreed on 13 responses over the classification (inter-rater reliability= 100%).

The responses of social workers of Astro Kids program to the three open-ended questions can be seen in Table 3. To enhance the reliability of the coding, a certain proportion of the responses for each question were randomly selected for inter-rater reliability checking. The findings suggest that the coding systems adopted were reliable.

It is noteworthy that most of the respondents perceived that the two most important things that participants of the Astro Kids program had learned from the program were drug knowledge and refusal skills (27% and 18% respectively). Most of them suggested that the program could be improved by reduction of activities that required writing and modification of some activities as stated in the manual (17% and 12 % respectively). The majority of them (70%) are willing to recommend the Astro Kids to other people.

SUBJECTIVE OUTCOMES BASED ON WORKERS OF THE ASTRO TEENS PROGRAM

The findings on the workers' evaluation (N=21) of the program details are shown in Table 4 and Table 5. As Table 4 shows, most were satisfied with the provision of information (95% were satisfied or very satisfied), arrangements of the day camp (81% were satisfied or very satisfied), provision of materials (95% were satisfied or very satisfied), workers' performance (95% were satisfied or very satisfied), refreshments (96% were satisfied or very satisfied), and arrangement of the program and other activities (81% and 48% were satisfied or very satisfied respectively). With regard to the perceived qualities of the program, most felt the program was good or very good with respect to the provision of information (95%), arrangements of the day camp (76%), provision of materials (86%), workers' performance (95%), refreshments (90%), and arrangement of the program (76%) and other activities (43%). It is evident that the qualities of the program activities were well received by most of the social workers.

Most of the workers felt that the program was either helpful or very helpful for adolescents in the areas of drug refusal attitudes (95%), improvement of drug refusal skills (81%), drug refusal behavior (90%), improvement of social skills (81%), and increase of drug knowledge (95%). The findings are displayed in Table 5. Similarly, most of the workers believed that the program could help group members refrain from smoking (52% of the responses were "Helpful"),

Table 4. Degree of satisfaction with and perceived qualities of the program amongst workers of the Astro Teens program (N=21)

	Level of Satisfaction					Perceived Qualities				
	Very Dis-satisfied	Dis-satisfied	Satisfied	Very Satisfied	Missing value	Very Poor	Poor	Good	Very Good	Missing Value
Information giving	0%	5%	76%	19%	0%	0%	0%	95%	0%	5%
Arrangement of day camp activities	0%	0%	52%	29%	19%	0%	0%	57%	19%	24%
Resources giving	0%	5%	81%	14%	0%	0%	10%	76%	10%	4%
Performance of workers	0%	5%	90%	5%	0%	0%	0%	95%	0%	5%
Refreshments	0%	0%	86%	10%	4%	0%	0%	80%	10%	10%
Arrangement of the program (e.g., place, activities, time, etc.)	0%	19%	67%	14%	0%	0%	19%	67%	9%	5%
Other activities	0%	9%	43%	5%	43%	0%	9%	38%	5%	48%

Table 5. Perceived helpfulness of the Astro Teens program by the workers (N=21)

	Not At All Helpful	Slightly Helpful	Helpful	Very Helpful
Attitude towards refusing drugs	0%	5%	71%	24%
Improvement of refusal skills towards drugs	0%	19%	62%	19%
Behavior on refusing drugs*	0%	5%	71%	19%
Improvement of social skills*	0%	14%	76%	5%
Enhancement of drug knowledge	0%	5%	57%	38%
Do you think "Astro Teens" program can help members to stay away from smoking?	5%	43%	52%	0%
Do you think "Astro Teens" program can help members to stay away from alcohol?	5%	48%	38%	9%
Do you think "Astro Teens" program can help members to stay away from drugs (e.g., Cannabis, Heroin, Ketamine, MDMA, "Ice")?	0%	5%	67%	28%
Do you think "Astro Teens" program can help members to prevent early sex?	0%	14%	62%	24%

*Missing value = 5%.

using alcohol and other drugs (47% and 95% of the responses were "Helpful" or "Very Helpful" respectively), and engaging in early sex (86% of the responses were "Helpful" or "Very Helpful").

The responses to the three open-ended questions can be seen in Table 6. To enhance the reliability of the coding, a certain proportion of the responses for each

Table 6. The responses of social workers of Astro Teens program to the open-ended questions

No.		Responses (N)	Percentage
a. Workers' perceptions of the most important things that participants of the Astro Teens program had learned from the program			
1	Drug knowledge	8	15%
2	Attitude towards refusing drugs	7	14%
3	Sex knowledge	5	10%
4	Awareness of the outcomes of abusing drugs	4	7%
5	Respecting other people	4	7%
6	Improving social skills	4	7%
7	Refusal skills	3	6%
8	Self understanding	3	6%
9	Coping with stress	3	6%
10	Listen to others	2	4%
11	Taking care of others	2	4%
12	Expressing personal view	2	4%
13	Awareness of the ingredients of gateway drugs	1	2%
14	Setting up goal	1	2%
15	Emotional control	1	2%
16	No comments	2	4%
Total		52	100%

No.		Responses (N)	Percentage
b. Workers' suggestions on how the Astro Teens program can be improved			
1	Reduction of the number of group sessions	6	20%
2	More game activities in each session	3	10%
3	Organizing overnight camp and adventure-based counseling activities	3	10%
4	Visits to drug rehabilitation organizations	2	7%
5	Linking sessions on gateway drugs and drug knowledge together	2	7%
6	Improvement of activities in role play sessions	1	4%
7	More practical emphasis and interaction in group activities	1	4%
8	Replace "Secret Angel" in each session by words that can express members' views	1	4%
9	Organizing more outdoor activities	1	4%
10	Reduction of the number of topics	1	4%
11	Reduction of the number of questionnaires	1	4%
12	Modifying worksheet of the last session	1	4%
13	Strengthening activities in the session on self-esteem	1	4%
14	No comments	4	14%
Total		28	100%

Table 6. (Continued)

No.		Responses (N)	Percentage
c. Workers' willingness to recommend the Astro Teens program to other people			
1	Yes	15	70%
2	Yes, for some sessions or if the manuals are revised	3	15%
3	No	1	5%
4	No comments	2	10%
Total		21	100%

Remarks:
a. Out of 15 randomly selected responses, the first rater and second rater agreed on 12 responses over the classification (inter-rater reliability= 80%).
b. Out of 10 randomly selected responses, the first rater and second rater agreed on 7 responses over the classification (inter-rater reliability= 70%).
c. Out of 10 randomly selected responses, the first rater and second rater agreed on 10 responses over the classification (inter-rater reliability= 100%).

question were randomly selected for inter-rater reliability checking. The findings suggest that the coding systems adopted were reliable. It is noteworthy that most of the respondents perceived that the two most important things that participants of the Astro Teens program had learned from the program were drug knowledge and attitude towards refusing drugs (15% and 14% respectively). Nearly one third of the respondents suggested that the program could be improved by reduction of the number of group sessions and having more game activities in each session (20% and 10% respectively). The majority of them (70%) are willing to recommend the Astro Teens to other people and the other 15% said that they would do so if the program could be slightly modified.

CONCLUSION

Overall, the subjective outcome evaluation data regarding the global evaluation of the Astro Teens and Astro Kids programs are generally positive, clearly indicated that most of the workers and participants(reported in another paper) were satisfied with the programs. As far as the social workers are concerned, they had perceived many positive features of the programs and agreed that the programs were helpful to the users in terms of healthy attitude formation, improvement of refusal skills towards drugs, behavior on refusing drugs, improvement of social skills, enhancement of drug knowledge, staying away from smoking, alcohol and drugs, and prevention of early sex (shown in Figures 1 and 2). In sum, the social workers were satisfied with the Astro programs in helping the participants in building resistance against substance abuse.

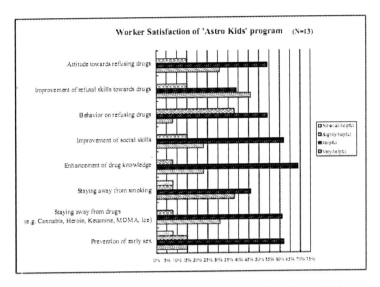

Figure 1. Client satisfaction findings based on the social workers (Astro Kids program).

Although it is common to receive high satisfaction rates in client satisfaction surveys (7), three points should be noted. First, two perspectives— those of the workers and the participants (refers to another paper) — were used in the survey, a practice which enables triangulation by data sources.

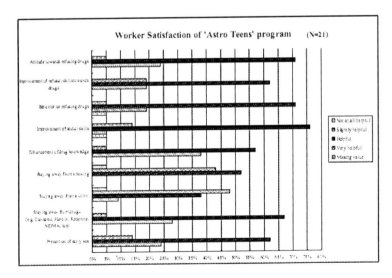

Figure 2. Client satisfaction findings based on the social workers (Astro Teens).

While it is common to explain high client satisfaction rates by demand characteristics, this is less likely to explain the high satisfaction rates among the social workers who were responsible for the implementation of Astro programs. Therefore, the use of two perspectives to look at client satisfaction data offers a more robust approach to assess subjective outcome measures. Second, because the identity of the workers and participants was concealed in the data collection process and there was no direct relationship between the authors (including our research assistants) and the respondents, the possibility of demand characteristics playing a role in this situation was not high. Finally, inter-rater reliability checking was carried out for the analyses of the open-ended questions and the findings suggest that the coding systems adopted were reliable.

While the subjective outcome data are very encouraging, there are two limitations of the present findings. First, in addition to using structured questions, more open-ended questions can be added to gain a more in-depth understanding of the experiences of the workers and participants. In particular, social workers can be asked to keep reflective journals about the program content, their observations and related experiences. Second, while evaluation instruments are used in the Western context, validation work in the Chinese context is needed. As pointed out by Royse (18), most of the available measures of subjective outcome assessment are "homemade." As a further step, validation of the related assessment tools in the Chinese context is necessary. This point is important because validated measures of subjective outcome measures of drug prevention are not currently available in Hong Kong. In fact, although many drug prevention programs for young people were launched, vigorous evaluation was almost non-existent in Hong Kong. In response to this unfortunate situation, Shek et al. (5,19) had developed the Project Astro, the pioneering drug prevention program, and the effectiveness of the related programs was vigorously evaluated. This effort has been a small step forward. In tackling the developmental challenges of the young people in a modern society, as pointed out by Shek (20,21), evidence-based intervention programs are one of the important things that we need, if we are going to face these challenges with them.

REFERENCES

[1] Peele S. The meaning of addiction – Compulsive experience and its interpretation. Lexington, MA: Lexington Books, 1985.
[2] Panter AT, Melchior L. Modeling the impact of school-based prevention on adolescent drug use. Score 1995;18:1-3.

[3] Stoil MJ, Hill G. Preventing substance abuse – Interventions that work. New York: Plenum, 1996.

[4] Hawkins JD, Catalano RE, Miller JY. Risk and protective factors for alcohol and other drug problems in adolescence and early adulthood: implications for substance use prevention. Psychol. Bull. 1992;112(1):64-105.

[5] Shek DTL, Ng HY, Lam CW, Lam OB, Yeung KC. A longitudinal evaluation study of a pioneering drug preventionprogram(Project Astro MIND) in Hong Kong. Hong Kong: Beat Drugs Fund and the Hong Kong Youth Institute, 2003.

[6] Holcomb WR, Adams NA, Ponder HM, Reitz R. The development and construction validation of a consumer satisfaction questionnaire for psychiatric patients. Eval. Program Plann.1989;12:189-94.

[7] Lebow JL. Research assessing consumer satisfaction with mental health treatment: areview of findings. Eval. Program Plann.1982;6:211-36.

[8] Lebow JL. Assessing consumer satisfaction in mental health treatment settings: aguide for the administrator. Adm.Ment. Health1984;12:3-14.

[9] McMurty SL, Hudson WW. The client satisfaction inventory: results of an initial validation study. Res.Soc. Work Pract.2000;10:644-63.

[10] Young SC, Nicholson J, Davis M. An overview of issues in research on consumer satisfaction with child and adolescent mental health services. J. Child Fam. Stud.1995;4:219-38.

[11] Ankuta G, Abeles N. Client satisfaction, clinical change and meaningful change in psychotherapy. Prof.Psychol.1993;24:70-4.

[12] Attkisson C, Zwick R. The client satisfaction questionnaire: psychometric properties and correlations with service utilization and psychotherapy outcome. Eval. Program Plann.1982;5:233-37.

[13] Carscaddon D, George M, Wells G. Rural community mental health consumer satisfaction and psychiatric symptoms. Community Ment. Health J.1990;26:309-18.

[14] Deane F. Client satisfaction with psychotherapy in two outpatient clinics in New Zealand. Eval. Program Plann.1993;16:87-94.

[15] Edwards D, Yarvis R, Mueller D, Langsley D. Does patient satisfaction correlate with success? Hosp. Community Psychiatry1978;29:188-90.

[16] Larsen D, Attkisson CC, Hargreaves WA, Nguyen TD. Assessment of client/patient satisfaction: development of a general scale.Eval. Program Plann.1979;2:197-207.

[17] LaSala MC. Client satisfaction: consideration of correlates and response bias. Fam. Soc. 1997;78(1):54-64.

[18] Royse D. Research methods in social work. Pacific Groves, CA: Brooks/Cole, 2004.

[19] Lam CW, Shek DTL, Ng HY, Yeung KC, Lam DOB. An innovation in drug prevention programs for adolescents: the Hong Kong Astro Project. Int. J. Adolesc. Med. Health 2005;17(4):343-53.

[20] Shek DTL. School drug testing: a critical review of the literature. Scientific World Journal 2010;10:356-65.

[21] Shek DTL. Enthusiasm-based or evidence-based charities: personal reflections based on the Project P.A.T.H.S. in Hong Kong. Scientific World Journal 2008;8:802-10.

In: Drug Abuse in Hong Kong
Editors: D Shek, R Sun and J Merrick
ISBN: 978-1-61324-491-3
©2012 Nova Science Publishers, Inc.

Chapter 7

THE QUALITATIVE EVALUATION OF THE PROGRAM PARTICIPANTS

Chiu-Wan Lam[1,a] and Daniel TL Shek[a,b,c,d,e]

[a]Department of Applied Social Sciences,
The Hong Kong Polytechnic University, Hong Kong, PRC
[b]Public Policy Research Institute,
The Hong Kong Polytechnic University, Hong Kong, PRC
[c]East China Normal University, Shanghai, PRC
[d]Kiang Wu Nursing College of Macau, Macau, PRC
[e]Division of Adolescent Medicine, Department of Pediatrics,
Kentucky Children's Hospital, University of Kentucky,
College of Medicine, Lexington, Kentucky, US

ABSTRACT

The subjective perceptions and personal experiences of the Astro program participants were explored by qualitative evaluation methods. A wide range of participants including those who experienced positive changes and those who did not, were recruited for a more comprehensive picture of their experiences. Questions regarding the participants' experiences of the project were asked. The in-depth interview data based on 30 participants

---

[1]Correspondence: Chiu-Wan Lam, MSW, PhD, Department of Applied Social Sciences, The Hong Kong Polytechnic University, Hong Kong. E-mail: sscwlam@polyu.edu.hk.

showed that their experiences with the program were very positive. They appreciated the unique characteristics of the program, observed positive changes in the program participants, and felt that the program was helpful to themselves and adolescents in general. If they could, most of the participants would join the program again.

INTRODUCTION

It is now well established in the drug prevention literature that drug information programs alone are ineffective. Worse still, the giving of information alone may increase drug use. For example, programs emphasizing the dangers of drug use may attract individuals who are sensation-seeking, whereas information about the chemical effects of drug may arouse the curiosity of those who may want to experience the psychoactive effects of these drugs, and telling people about the modes of administration and other details of drug use may become a brief course on drug use rather than on preventing drug use (1). Recent approaches have turned to focus on comprehensive strategies that target early risk factors in adolescent drug use. These factors include: a) individual risk factors like poor social skills, low self-esteem, and favorable attitudes towards drug use, and b) environmental risk factors like a family environment with poor parent-child bonding, or low parental involvement in their children. Association with drug-using peers, however, is even more conducive to drug use than family influence. Drug use is also found to correlate with poor school performance and delinquent behavior (2).

In McNeal and Hansen's (3) longitudinal study of the key mediators for adolescent drug use, they identified deterioration in four specific mediators as most related to the onset of drug use: normative beliefs (peer beliefs and endorsement of drug use), manifest commitment (not to use drugs), lifestyle incompatibility with drug use, and beliefs about consequences of drug use. They recommend future research to focus on variables that are most significant for explaining drug use.

Based on the above observations, effective drug prevention work should seek to eliminate environmental influences which promote or facilitate drug use, and at the same time, reduce adolescents' vulnerability to the various environmental factors promoting drug use, given that drug abuse occurs as a result of both environmental and individual factors (4). Hawkins et al. (5) have specifically asked for a risk-focused approach to drug prevention that seeks to reduce or buffer the effects of known antecedents of adolescent drug abuse, i.e., the cultivation of protective factors in high-risk youth. These include parenting skills, social competence abilities training, youth involvement in alternative activities and comprehensive risk-focused programs. The adaptation of programs in the Project Astrois obviously consistent with the spirit of a risk-focused approach.

OUR PROJECT

The subjective perceptions and personal experiences of program participants can are explored by qualitative evaluation methods, though quantitative evaluation can provide insight into group differences (6-11). According to Denzin and Lincoln (12-15), there is different schools of qualitative inquiry. In the present evaluation, rather than following a single qualitative approach (such as a grounded theory approach or a phenomenological approach), general principles in qualitative research were adopted. First, open-ended interview questions without preset answers were used and the participants could freely narrate in the interviews. Second, the subjective viewpoints and experiences of the participants were respected. Third, in-depth collection of information was carried out. Fourth, an inductive approach was used so that the themes and patterns of responses could emerge from the data. Fifth, the researchers were aware of the possibility of biases and preoccupation in the data collection and analyses processes. Finally, inter-rater reliability checks were carried out.

Although they were recruited via convenient sampling, a wide range of participants, including those who experienced positive changes and those who did not, were recruited for a more comprehensive picture of their experiences. The questions of the interview schedule were modeled after the CIPP model (16,17). A semi-structured interview guide regarding product (outcomes) evaluation of the program was developed. The primary function of product evaluation is to measure, interpret, and judge a program's successes (17). As such, evaluation questions that determine the extent to which identified needs were met and the identification of the broad effects of the program were asked.

Questions regarding the participants' experiences of the project were asked (17). The following questions were included in the interview guide:

a. Overall, what views do you have of the program?
b. What do you think are the special features of this group?
c. Do you like the group format? Why or why not?
d. What are your views regarding the content of the group?
e. Which group session(s) did you find the most memorable?

f. Did the group leave you with any lasting impressions?
g. How would you describe your interaction with the group members?
h. How would you describe your interaction with the group leader?
i. What were your initial experiences with the group?
j. What were your experiences after joining the group?
k. What changes did you experience after joining the group?(Your knowledge of drugs? Attitude toward drugs? Experience with drugs? Your knowledge of sex?Attitude toward sex?Sexual experience?Your mentality?Interaction with others? Relationship with family members?)
l. If you experienced changes after joining the program, what factors contributed to these changes?
m. If you did not experience changes after joining the program, what factors contributed to the lack of changes?
n. Do you think this group is helpful to young people?
o. What changes are needed for this group?
p. If you could, would you join this group again? Why or why not?
q. Were you satisfied with this group? Were there any areas that you were dissatisfied with?

OUR FINDINGS

The content of the interviews for the program participants (N=30) was transcribed. To facilitate analyses, a pre-structured case approach with reference to the interview questions or areas of interview questions was adopted (18). Our unit of analysis was a meaningful unit instead of a statement. For example, the statement "the program helps me gain more knowledge on substance abuse and develop more positive attitudes towards substance abuse" would be broken down to two meaningful units or attributes, namely, "the program helps me gain more knowledge on substance abuse" and "the program helps me develop more positive attitudes towards drug abuse" (19,20). To examine the reliability of the coding schemes for some of the questions (particularly those regarding the effectiveness and benefits of the program), some of the protocols were randomly selected and coded by another rater to generate measures of inter-rater reliability (i.e., triangulation by researchers).

Regarding the views of the participants(N=30)toward the group, the responses were generally positive. In addition to having fun, some of the participants reported experiencing positive changes after joining the group. The relevant findings are presented in Table 1a. When the participants were asked

Table 1. Participants' responses to the qualitative interview

No.	Items	Responses (N)	Percentage
\multicolumn{4}{l}{a. Question: "What are your feelings and views towards the group?"}
1	Having fun and enjoyment	14	41.18%
2	Quite good	8	23.53%
3	Could learn much knowledge	6	17.65%
4	Cohesive	2	5.88%
5	Happy	2	5.88%
6	Seeing changes in myself	1	2.94%
7	The program was helpful	1	2.94%
	Total	34	100%
\multicolumn{4}{l}{b. Question: "What do you think are the special features about the group?"}
1	Sent the messages through discussion and activities	10	29.42%
2	Could learn much knowledge through games	8	23.53%
3	Provided much knowledge to participants	3	8.83%
4	Cultivated group cohesion through activities	2	5.88%
5	No fixed rules	2	5.88%
6	Learned from the outdoor activities and training in "Astro Leaders" program (e.g., camping, hip-pop dancing)	2	5.88%
7	Relationships with workers and members became close	1	2.94%
8	Focused on the knowledge and effects of drug abuse	1	2.94%
9	Discussion of the future life with group members	1	2.94%
10	No special feature	4	11.76%
	Total	34	100%

Remarks:
a. Out of 20 randomly selected responses, the first rater and second rater agreed on 16 responses over the classification (inter-rater reliability = 80%).
b. Out of 20 randomly selected responses, the first rater and second rater agreed on 15 responses over the classification (inter-rater reliability = 75%).

about the special features of the group, they mentioned several elements, including learning via discussion and activities, use of games, and cultivation of group cohesion (Table 1b).

Concerning the participants' perceptions of the content of the group, the responses were generally positive. Roughly one-fourth of the responses were negative about the format of the groups and six responses were "no comment" (Table 2).

Table 2. Participants' responses to the question "what do you think about the content of the group?"

No.	Items	Responses (N)	Percentage
	Positive Responses:		
1	Quite good	6	19.35%
2	Different topics were helpful to group members	2	6.45%
3	Knowledge transmitted through games and activities	2	6.45%
4	The use of group format was impressive	2	6.45%
5	The games were interesting	2	6.45%
6	Discussion and sharing sessions were interesting	2	6.45%
7	Learned more about the harmful effects of smoking and drinking	1	3.23%
	Negative Responses:		
8	Some games were boring	5	16.14%
9	Some of the topics were the same and repetitive	2	6.45%
10	Repetitive formats in the Questions and Answers competitions	1	3.23%
11	No comment	6	19.35%
	Total	31	100%

Remarks:
i. Out of 20 randomly selected responses, the first rater and second rater agreed on 16 responses over the categorization in terms of the basic categories (inter-rater reliability = 80%).
ii. Out of 20 randomly selected responses, the first rater and second rater agreed on 18 responses over the classification of positive and negative responses (inter-rater reliability = 90%).

Regarding the experiences of the participants at the initial phase of the program, more than half of the responses were either neutral or negative. These respondents either had no expectations or felt that they were forced by the school to join. On the other hand, 33.3% of the responses were positive, relating to the participants' expectations about joining the program. The findings are presented in Table 3. However, when the participants were asked about their experiences after joining the group, nearly all responses were positive, with only two respondents not reporting any differences after joining the group (Table 3).

Table 3. Participants' responses to the qualitative interview

No.	Items	Responses (N)	Percentage
a. Question: "What are your expectations and feelings when joining the group at the beginning?"			
	Positive Responses:		
1	Expected to play	6	18.18%
2	Desired to learn, such as knowledge about drugs	3	9.09%
3	Wished to be more independent and confident of myself	1	3.03%

The qualitative evaluation of the program participants 107

No.	Items	Responses (N)	Percentage
4	Wished to learn the ways of reducing stress	1	3.03%
	Neutral Responses:		
5	No expectation	12	36.37%
6	No expectation because forced by the school to join	7	21.21%
	Negative Responses:		
7	Much resistance as I was labeled "bad student" by the teacher	3	9.09%
	Total	33	100%
	b. Question: "What are your feelings after joining the group?"		
1	Fruitful such as gaining knowledge about drug and sex	9	23.68%
2	Quite good and enjoyable	7	18.42%
3	Happier than expected	4	10.54%
4	Would like to join the group again	4	10.54%
5	Changes in myself	2	5.26%
6	Increased sense of belonging to the group	2	5.26%
7	My relationships with friends and others have improved	2	5.26%
8	Have learned interpersonal skills and cooperation with others	1	2.63%
9	Have learned independence and confidence	1	2.63%
10	Abilities of oneself validated by group activities	1	2.63%
11	Have had greater sense of responsibility	1	2.63%
12	Have begun to be more considerate to others	1	2.63%
13	Was able to take part in voluntary service	1	2.63%
14	No differences when compared with the beginning phase of the group	2	5.26%
	Total	38	100%

Remarks:
i. Out of 20 randomly selected responses, the first rater and second rater agreed on 14 responses over the categorization in terms of the basic categories (inter-rater reliability = 70%).
ii. Out of 20 randomly selected responses, the first rater and second rater agreed on 16 responses over the classification of positive and negative responses (inter-rater reliability = 80%).
iii. Out of 25 randomly selected responses, the first rater and second rater agreed on 22 responses over the classification (inter-rater reliability = 88%).

Table 4. Participants' responses to the question "what are your changes after joining the program?"

No.	Content	Responses (N)	Percentage
	a. Drug knowledge		
	Positive Responses:		
1	Learned more about drugs	26	70.27%
2	Learned the harmful effects and consequences of drug abuse	3	8.11%
3	Learned more about cigarette and its ingredients	2	5.41%
4	Learned more about refusal skills	2	5.41%
	Neutral Responses:		
5	No changes	4	10.80%
	Total	37	100%

Table 4. (Continued)

No.	Content	Responses (N)	Percentage
b. Attitude towards Drugs			
Positive Responses:			
1	Less favorable attitudes to drugs and more thoughts about the consequences	7	24.13%
2	Less curious about drugs after joining the program	5	17.24%
3	Held a more serious attitude towards drugs and would not try in a casual manner	4	13.79%
4	Would not take drugs because of bad mood	3	10.34%
5	Would not take drugs because of peer influence	1	3.45%
6	Attitude changed from "does not really matter" to "definitely will not try"	1	3.45%
Neutral Responses:			
7	No changes as I would not take drugs	7	24.13%
8	No changes	1	3.45%
Total		29	100%
c. Behavioral intention towards Drugs			
Positive Responses:			
1	No more drugs attempts after joining the group	21	58.33%
2	Took less drugs when compared with the past	4	11.11%
3	Would tell others about the harmful effect of drugs abuse	3	8.33%
4	Took Ecstasy before, but absolutely would not take now	2	5.56%
5	Smoked less because it is harmful to our lungs	1	2.78%
Neutral Responses:			
6	No changes	5	13.89%
Total		36	100%
d. Sex knowledge			
Positive Responses:			
1	Learned more about sex	18	40.91%
2	Learned more about refusal skills in sex	9	20.45%
3	Learned more about the consequences of sexual intercourse	3	6.82%
4	Learned more about the legal issues around sex	2	4.55%
Neutral Responses:			
5	No changes	12	27.27%
Total		44	100%
e. Attitude towards sex			
Positive Responses:			
1	More positive when talking about sex rather than feeling embarrassed	9	25.71%
2	Would think more about the outcome of sexual intercourse	5	14.29%
3	Would not attempt	1	2.86%
Neutral Responses:			
4	No changes	20	57.14%
Total		35	100%
f. Behavioral intention towards sex			
Positive Responses:			

The qualitative evaluation of the program participants

No.	Content	Responses (N)	Percentage
1	Would not have sexual intercourse with others casually	5	16.67%
2	Would not try	6	20.00%
3	Would set an age limit for myself	1	3.33%
	Neutral Responses:		
4	No changes and would say "no"	9	30.00%
5	No changes	9	30.00%
	Total	30	100%
	g. Changes of self		
	Positive Responses:		
1	Became more optimistic	6	17.65%
2	Better self-knowledge	6	17.65%
3	Better emotional control	5	14.72%
4	Became psychologically stronger	3	8.82%
5	Knew different ways to solve problems	2	5.88%
6	Knew how to accept others' views	2	5.88%
7	Became more enthusiastic	2	5.88%
8	Knew how to reduce stress	1	2.94%
9	Increase in self-confidence	1	2.94%
10	Increase in sense of responsibility	1	2.94%
11	Knew how to express one's views	1	2.94%
	Neutral Responses:		
12	No changes	4	11.76%
	Total	34	100%
	h. Human relationship		
	Positive Responses:		
1	Learned how to communicate with others	8	26.67%
2	Learned how to accommodate and concern others	4	13.33%
3	Relationship with teachers became better and improved	4	13.33%
4	Learned how to respect others	1	3.34%
	Neutral Responses:		
5	No changes	3	10.00%
6	The question was not asked in the interview	10	33.33%
	Total	30	100%
	i. Relationship with the family		
	Positive Responses:		
1	Relationship has improved	9	29.04%
2	More communication with parents	2	6.45%
3	More understanding of the feelings of family members	2	6.45%
4	Learned how to respect family members	1	3.23%
	Neutral Responses:		
5	No change	11	35.48%
6	The question was not asked in the interviews	6	19.35%
	Total	31	100%

Remarks:
a. Out of 20 randomly selected responses, the first rater and second rater agreed on 16 responses over the categorization in terms of the basic categories (inter-rater reliability = 80%).

Table 4. (Continued)

b. Out of 20 randomly selected responses, the first rater and second rater agreed on 18 responses over the classification of positive and negative responses (inter-rater reliability = 90%).

c. Out of 20 randomly selected responses, the first rater and second rater agreed on 14 responses over the categorization in terms of the basic categories (inter-rater reliability = 70%). Out of 20 randomly selected responses, the first rater and second rater agreed on 16 responses over the classification of positive and negative responses (inter-rater reliability = 80%).

d. Out of 25 randomly selected responses, the first rater and second rater agreed on 22 responses over the categorization in terms of the basic categories (inter-rater reliability = 88%). Out of 25 randomly selected responses, the first rater and second rater agreed on 23 responses over the classification of positive and negative responses (inter-rater reliability = 92%).

e. Out of 25 randomly selected responses, the first rater and second rater agreed on 20 responses over the categorization in terms of the basic categories (inter-rater reliability = 80%). Out of 25 randomly selected responses, the first rater and second rater agreed on 22 responses over the classification of positive and negative responses (inter-rater reliability = 88%).

f. Out of 20 randomly selected responses, the first rater and second rater agreed on 17 responses over the categorization in terms of the basic categories (inter-rater reliability = 85%). Out of 20 randomly selected responses, the first rater and second rater agreed on 18 responses over the classification of positive and negative responses (inter-rater reliability = 90%).

g. Out of 20 randomly selected responses, the first rater and second rater agreed on 14 responses over the categorization in terms of the basic categories (inter-rater reliability = 70%). Out of 20 randomly selected responses, the first rater and second rater agreed on 17 responses over the classification of positive and negative responses (inter-rater reliability = 85%).

h. Out of 25 randomly selected responses, the first rater and second rater agreed on 22 responses over the categorization in terms of the basic categories (inter-rater reliability = 88%). Out of 25 randomly selected responses, the first rater and second rater agreed on 23 responses over the classification of positive and negative responses (inter-rater reliability = 92%).

i. Out of 15 randomly selected responses, the first rater and second rater agreed on 12 responses over the categorization in terms of the basic categories (inter-rater reliability = 80%). Out of 15 randomly selected responses, the first rater and second rater agreed on 13 responses over the classification of positive and negative responses (inter-rater reliability = 86.67%).

j. Out of 15 randomly selected responses, the first rater and second rater agreed on 11 responses over the categorization in terms of the basic categories (inter-rater reliability = 73.33%). Out of 15 randomly selected responses, the first rater and second rater agreed on 13 responses over the classification of positive and negative responses (inter-rater reliability = 86.67%).

Concerning the participants' perceptions of the changes after joining the group, the findings generally suggested that the program was effective. In the area of drug knowledge, only 4 out of 37 responses were neutral, with most suggesting that the participants acquired drug knowledge from the program (Table 4a). Regarding drug attitudes, with the exception of eight responses that were neutral (i.e., attitudes did not change after joining the program), all the responses suggested that the participants improved their attitudes (Table 4b). Most of the responses in Table 4c also suggested that the participants were less likely to take drugs after joining the program.

With respect to sex knowledge, the findings presented in Table 4d show that the majority of the participants felt they had learned more about sex. Concerning willingness to abstain from sex, the positive responses represent roughly half of the total responses (Table 4e and Table 4f, respectively).

An examination of the findings in Table 4g shows that the program had positive changes on most of the program participants. With the exception of four neutral responses (i.e., no personal changes reported after joining the program), all the responses were positive. There is also evidence indicating that the participants' relationships with their families and other people improved after joining the program (Table 4h and i).

When asked whether they would like to join the program again, a majority of the participants indicated they would (Table 5a). In addition to viewing the program as helpful to themselves, the participants felt it would be helpful to adolescents in general. Out of 31 responses summarized in Table 5b, only two reported that the program was not helpful to adolescents. Finally, the participants' views on how the program could be improved are summarized in Table 5c. Their suggestions were mainly related to the format and content of the group sessions.

The positive effects of the program can be seen in the following narratives of the participants:

Table 5. Participants' responses to the qualitative interview

No.	Items	Responses (N)	Percentage
a. Question: "Would you take part in the group again if you were given a chance? Why?"			
	Yes:		
1	Enjoyable	12	38.71%
2	Can learn much such as the knowledge on drugs and sex	3	9.68%
3	Would join if new topics were introduced	2	6.45%
4	Can learn more about oneself	2	6.45%
5	Joyful experiences	2	6.45%
6	Helpful to oneself	1	3.23%
7	No reason	6	19.35%
	No:		
8	No reason	3	9.68%
	Total	31	100%
b. Question: "Do you think this group is helpful to the adolescents?"			
	Yes:		
1	No explanation offered	10	32.25%
2	Particular helpful for young people to learn different kinds of knowledge, such as topics on drug abuse, sex and self-exploration	9	29.01%
3	Helpful to docile adolescents	3	9.67%
4	Can learn and apply refusal skills	1	3.23%
5	Helpful to those members who live in the hostel	1	3.23%
6	Helpful to those members who join the program for the first time	1	3.23%
7	Helpful because the topics are very appropriate to contemporary	1	3.23%

No.	Items	Responses (N)	Percentage
	young people		
8	Can help young people to deal with their rebellious emotion	1	3.23%
9	Can cultivate team spirit among members	1	3.23%
10	Provides another alternative for young people	1	3.23%
	No:		
11	Not helpful to non-hostel members as they only play and would not have time to think about themselves	1	3.23%
12	Hard to change the beliefs of adolescents, especially those who are drug abusers	1	3.23%
Total		31	100%
c. Question: "What improvements would you like to make for the group?"			
1	More active forms of activities other than discussion and written exercises	9	19.15%
2	More outdoor activities, such as camping, hiking, playing war game	7	14.88%
3	Shorter time duration	5	10.64%
4	More involvement of members in the group	2	4.25%
5	Insufficient time for the group, can be better improved by extending half an hour in the group	2	4.25%
6	Can invite ex-drug abusers to share their experiences	2	4.25%
7	Workers can give more encouragement to members to involve more in the groups	1	2.13%
8	Workers can have more communication with staff in the center	1	2.13%
9	Some activities can be simplified, such as the activity of blowing balloons in the second session, so that workers can bring out the objectives of the activities easily	1	2.13%
10	Improve the timing for bringing out the objectives of the activities since members would not respond positively after the activities	1	2.13%
11	Pay more attention to the willingness of the members to join the group when recruiting group members	1	2.13%
12	Add a revision session after finishing every 3 sessions so that members can revise what they have learned	1	2.13%
13	Can add some sessions related to the interests of young people (e.g., sessions on playing guitar and basketball)	1	2.13%
14	Broadcast anti-drug video tapes in the group	1	2.13%
15	More refreshments and prizes	1	2.13%
16	Increase the number of sessions	1	2.13%
17	Reduce the number of posttest measures	1	2.13%
18	No, because everything was quite good	9	19.15%
Total		47	100%

Remarks:

a. Out of 20 randomly selected responses, the first rater and second rater agreed on 18 responses over the classification (inter-rater reliability = 90%).

b. Out of 25 randomly selected responses, the first rater and second rater agreed on 21 responses over the classification (inter-rater reliability = 84%).

c. Out of 30 randomly selected responses, the first rater and second rater agreed on 26 responses over the classification (inter-rater reliability = 86.67%).

Participant 1 (Astro Kids program)

"I was a little bit resistant to drugs in the past, but my resistance is even greater now. With my increased knowledge, I understand the severity of taking drugs. I don't even smoke now."

Participant 2 (Astro Kids program)

"After joining the group, relationships between teachers and members improved. In the past, I spoke bad language in school and the teachers always scolded me. But my relationship with the teachers is better now and they even praise me."

Participant 3 (Astro Teens program)

"I have a deeper understanding about drugs, especially the harmful effects of MDMA and ketamine. After listening to the workers, I started to take fewer drugs and become more concerned about my health problems, such as memory loss and hand tremors as a result of taking ketamine and MDMA. Actually, I feel worse after getting 'high.'"

Participant 4 (Astro Teens program)

"I have changed. I am not exactly a substance abuser and have only tried drugs once or twice. In the past, I had given up. I knew that drugs might cost me my life. But now I don't use drugs anymore because I know it is not a good thing. If a person does not get killed, he or she will suffer other consequences that are really terrible and painful."

DISCUSSION

The in-depth interview data based on 30 participants showed that the participants' experiences with the program were very positive. They appreciated the unique characteristics of the program, perceived positive changes in themselves after they joined it, and felt that the program was helpful to themselves and adolescents in general. If they could, most of the participants would join the program again. Finally, some areas for improvement were suggested. Moreover, perceptions of the workers (reported in another paper) and participants were quite consistent regarding the unique features of the program and its positive impact.

Three features of the qualitative evaluation findings make them credible. First, the collection of the perspectives of the social workers (reported in another paper) and program participants enables us to have a triangulation of data sources. Second, a substantial number of social workers (N=15) and participants (N=30) were recruited to participate in the in-depth interviews. Although the participants were not randomly selected, the diversity of the participants recruited generated a fairly comprehensive picture of the participants' perceptions of the program and its effectiveness. Third, inter-rater reliability checking was carried out, particularly with respect to questions about the benefits of the program and changes in the participants after joining it.

Although experimental and quantitative approaches are commonly used to evaluate program effectiveness, it is argued that it is important to adopt a qualitative approach to explore the clients' positive and negative experiences of services and their perceptions of the improvement of services that could be made. Other researchers also support for the use of qualitative research methods to elicit the clients' subjective experiences and perceptions of services, in order to complement the quantitative findings on client satisfaction and to yield valuable information about the functioning of the services (21). For example, in the Project P.A.T.H.S. in Hong Kong, qualitative data were collected to illuminate the subjective experiences of the program participants and implementers (22,23). Obviously, these studies provide very good examples on how qualitative evaluation could be conducted in the Chinese contexts.

REFERENCES

[1] Panter AT, Melchior L. Modeling the impact of school-based prevention on adolescent drug use. Score 1995;18:1-3.
[2] Glantz M. A developmental psychopathology model of drug abuse vulnerability. In: Glantz M, Pickens R. Vulnerability to drug abuse. Washington, DC: Am. Psychol. Assoc. 1992:389-418.
[3] McNeal JrR, Hansen WB. Developmental patterns associated with the onset of drug use: changes in postulated mediators during adolescence. J. Drug. Issues 1999;29(2):381-400.

[4] Stoil MJ, Hill G. Preventing substance abuse – Interventions that work. New York: Plenum, 1996.
[5] Hawkins JD, Catalano RE, Miller JY. Risk and protective factors for alcohol and other drug problems in adolescence and early adulthood: implications for substance use prevention. Psychol. Bull. 1992;112(1):64-105.
[6] Berg BL. Qualitative research methods for the social sciences. Boston, MA: Allyn Bacon, 2003.
[7] Bryman A. Quantity and quality in social research. London: Unwin Hyman, 1988.
[8] MinichielloV. In-depth interviewing: Researching people. Melbourne: Longman Cheshire, 1990.
[9] Neuman WL, Kreuger LW. Social work research methods: Qualitative and quantitative approaches. Boston, MA: Allyn Bacon, 2003.
[10] Lincoln YS, Guba EG. Naturalistic inquiry. Beverly Hills, CA: Sage, 1985.
[11] Patton MQ. Qualitative research and evaluation methods.Thousand Oaks, CA: Sage, 2002.
[12] Denzin K, Lincoln, YS. The landscape of qualitative research. Thousand Oaks, CA: Sage, 1998.
[13] Denzin K, Lincoln, YS. Strategies of qualitative inquiry.Thousand Oaks, CA: Sage, 1998.
[14] Denzin K, Lincoln, YS. Collecting and interpreting qualitative materials.Thousand Oaks, CA: Sage, 1998.
[15] Denzin K, Lincoln, YS. Handbook of qualitative research.Thousand Oaks, CA: Sage, 2000.
[16] Stufflebeam DL. The CIPP model for evaluation. In: Stufflebeam DL, Medaus GF, Kellaghan T. eds.Evaluation models: Viewpoints on educational and human services evaluation. Boston, MA: Kluwer, 2000:279-318.
[17] Stufflebeam D, Shinkfeld AJ. Systematic evaluation. Boston, MA: Kluwer-Nijhoff, 1985.
[18] Miles MB, Huberman A. An expanded sourcebook:Qualitative data analysis. Newbury Park, CA: Sage, 1994.
[19] Shek DTL. Chinese adolescents and their parents' views on a happy family: implications for family therapy. Fam. Ther. 2001;28:73-103.
[20] Shek DTL, Chan LK. Perceptions of the ideal child in a Chinese context. J.Psychol. 1999;133(3):291-302.
[21] Shek DTL, Ng CSM.Qualitative evaluation of the Project P.A.T.H.S.: findings based on focus groups with student participants. Scientific World Journal 2009;9:691-703.
[22] Shek DTL, Sun RCF, Tang CYP. Focus group evaluation from the perspective of program implementers: findings based on the Secondary 2 Program. Scientific World Journal 2009;9:992-1002.
[23] Shek DTL, Ng CSM, Tsui PF. Qualitative evaluation of the Project P.A.T.H.S.: findings based on focus groups.Int. J. Disabil. Hum. Dev. 2010;9(4):307-13.

In: Drug Abuse in Hong Kong
Editors: D Shek, R Sun and J Merrick
ISBN: 978-1-61324-491-3
©2012 Nova Science Publishers, Inc.

Chapter 8

THE PERSPECTIVE OF THE PROGRAM IMPLEMENTERS

Daniel TL Shek[1,a,b,c,d,e] *and Chiu-Wan Lam*[a]

[a]Department of Applied Social Sciences,
The Hong Kong Polytechnic University, Hong Kong, PRC
[b]Public Policy Research Institute,
The Hong Kong Polytechnic University, Hong Kong, PRC
[c]East China Normal University, Shanghai, PRC
[d]Kiang Wu Nursing College of Macau, Macau, PRC
[e]Division of Adolescent Medicine, Department of Pediatrics,
Kentucky Children's Hospital, University of Kentucky,
College of Medicine, Lexington, Kentucky, US

ABSTRACT

A total of 15 workers implementing the Astro Kid and Astro Teens programs in Hong Kong participated in qualitative evaluation interviews after completion of the programs. Interview questions were designed around the CIPP model, focusing on the evaluation of the context, input, process, and product of the programs. Results showed that the workers had positive

---

[1] Correspondence: Professor Daniel TL Shek, PhD, FHKPS, BBS, JP, Chair Professor, Department of Applied Social Sciences, The Hong Kong Polytechnic University, Hunghom, Hong Kong. E-mail: daniel.shek@polyu.edu.hk.

perceptions of the different aspects of the programs, particularly the process and product of the programs. The findings generally showed that the program implementers had positive perceptions of the programs and they perceived that the programs were able to protect the participants from substance abuse.

INTRODUCTION

In Hong Kong there is an increasing concern about the problem behavior of contemporary youth due to a steady rise in youth participation in and severity of substance abuse (1). To put these problems in context, for instance, a recent local study with community samples investigated substance abuse among secondary school students found that the lifetime prevalence of substance abuse has increased in recent years (2). Youth workers, youth development experts, social workers, program funders, program implementers, and researchers who study adolescent development have increasingly come to believe that prevention is better than cure. Therefore, there is a need to explore adolescent drug prevention programs. Nevertheless, there is a severe lack of adolescent drug prevention programs in Hong Kong.

In view of the severe lack of systematic and documented drug prevention programs in Hong Kong, the authors and their colleagues developed a pioneering drug prevention program – the Astro program (3, 4). The Astro program is a psychosocial primary prevention program for high-risk youth, focusing on peer and other influences on youth to use drugs, and on the development of skills to resist those temptations. It consists of three sequential and developmentally appropriate programs starting in early adolescence, with each program conducted in the form of structured group sessions. Apart from providing drug information, the content of the sessions also deals with themes relevant to adolescent development such as puberty and friendship. The related programs also teach young people a broad range of social and personal competences and help them to identify and deal with peer and other social pressures, to avoid drug uses, and to resist engaging in early sexual activities.

According to Patton (5), there are two main approaches in the field of evaluation, the quantitative/experimental approach and the qualitative/naturalistic approach. The quantitative/experimental paradigm has the following features: quantitative data (use of numbers and statistics), experimental designs, use of treatment and control groups, deductive hypothesis testing, objective perspective, evaluator aloof from the program, independent and dependent variables, linear and sequential modeling, pre-post focus on change, probabilistic and random sampling, standardized and uniform procedures, fixed and controlled designs, statistical analysis, emphasis on objective measurement, and generalizations. On the other hand, the qualitative/naturalistic paradigm possesses the following attributes: qualitative data (e.g., narratives and observations), naturalistic inquiry, case studies, inductive analysis, subjective perspective, evaluator close to the program, holistic contextual portrayal, systems perspective focused on interdependencies, dynamic and ongoing view of change, purposeful sampling of relevant cases, focus on uniqueness and diversity, emergent and flexible designs, thematic content analysis, and extrapolations (6). An examination of the field of prevention shows that although there is still a strong preference for the use of the quantitative/experimental approach to evaluate the effectiveness of prevention programs for adolescents, the number of qualitative evaluation studies in this area is increasing.

While quantitative evaluation can give ideas about group differences, qualitative studies can help to understand the subjective perceptions and personal experiences of the participants. According to Denzin and Lincoln (7), there are different branches in qualitative inquiry. In the present evaluation, instead of following a single qualitative approach (such as grounded theory approach or phenomenological approach), general principles in qualitative research were adopted. First, open-ended interview questions without preset answers were used and the informants could freely narrate in the interviews. Second, the subjective viewpoints and experiences of the informants were respected. Third, in-depth collection of information was carried out. Fourth, an inductive approach was used so that the themes and patterns of responses could emerge from the data. Fifth, the researchers were conscious of the possibilities of biases and preoccupation in the data collection and analyses processes. Finally, inter-rater reliability checks were carried out.

The purpose of this paper is to describe some of the qualitative findings based on focus group interviews with workers implementing the Astro Kids and Astro Teens programs. Although there are many strands of qualitative research (7), the most commonly used approach is the general qualitative approach where the general strategies of qualitative research are employed (e.g., collection of qualitative data, respecting the views of the informants, data analysis without preset coding scheme) but a specific qualitative approach is not adhered to (5). The exposition of the nature of this qualitative study is consistent with the view of Shek, Han, and Tang (6) that there should be an explicit statement of the philosophical base of the study (Principle 1).

OUR PROJECT

A total of 15 workers implementing the Astro Kids and Astro Teens programs were recruited and in-depth interviews were carried out to gain an understanding of their experiences and perceived benefits of the program as well as their perceived changes in the participants after joining the program. Although the workers were recruited via convenient sampling, a wide range of workers from different agencies and schools were recruited so that we could have a more comprehensive picture about the subjective experiences of the workers. The questions of the interview schedule were modeled after the CIPP model (8, 9). A semi-structured interview guide regarding context (planning decisions), input (structuring decisions), process (implementation decisions), and product (outcomes) evaluation of the program were examined.

As far as *context evaluation* is concerned, the workers' views on the context of evaluation, such as the needs of the participants as well as the strengths and weaknesses of the available programs were collected. Some of the questions are as follows:

- Have you conducted any drug prevention program before? If yes, for how many times?
- What were the training methods in the previous drug prevention programs?
- Did you carry out any evaluation for the previous drug prevention programs? How was it done?
- Were the previous prevention programs effective?
- How much do you know about Project Astro MIND?
- There are many structured drug prevention programs in the West. Do you have any understanding of such program?

For *input evaluation*, questions related to the appropriate approaches intended to bring about changes and the structural plans were asked (9). The questions in the interview guide included:

- How did you choose the program participants?
- Did your involvement in this project affect your regular work?
- Did you receive adequate support for the implementation of the program?
- What was the situation regarding the collaboration among the school, agency and community?

The perspective of the program implementers

Regarding *process evaluation*, questions regarding the actual implementation of the project, including its strengths and weaknesses, were asked (9). The questions in the interview guide included:

- Did you have any specific experiences regarding the implementation of the group?
- Did you experience any difficulties?
- What are your views on the applicability of the project? Was it user-friendly?
- What are your views on the different sessions of the program?
- What are your feelings regarding the responses of the members to the program?
- What are your responses to the project?
- What are your views on the evaluation of the project?
- Do you have any views on the routines of collaboration?

The primary function of *product evaluation* is "to measure, interpret, and judge the attainments of a program" (9, p.176). As such, evaluation questions that determine the extent to which identified needs were met and the identification of the broad effects of the program were asked:

- What is your impression about the project?
- What do you think are the uniqueness of the project?
- Do you think the project has influences on the members? If yes, what do you think are the factors that lead to such effects?
- What do you think are the changes in the members after they joined the program?
  - Knowledge, attitude, and behavior regarding drugs?
  - Knowledge, attitude, and behavior regarding sex?
- Are there any other aspects of change on members?
- What do you think about the effectiveness of the project?
- What do you think are the differences between this project and other similar projects?
- Which areas in the program are needed to be changed?

OUR FINDINGS

The content of the interviews with the workers (N=15) was transcribed. To facilitate analyses, a pre-structured case approach with reference to the interview questions or areas of interview questions was adopted (10). Our unit of analysis was a meaningful unit instead of a statement. For example, the statement that "the program helps me to gain more knowledge on substance abuse and develop more positive attitudes to avoid substance abuse" would be broken down to two meaningful units or attributes, namely, "the program helps me to gain more knowledge on substance abuse" and "the program helps me to develop more positive attitudes to avoid drug abuse" (11, 12). To examine the reliability of the coding schemes for some of the questions (particularly those questions regarding the effectiveness and benefits of the program), a certain proportion of the protocols were randomly selected and coded by another rater to generate measures of inter-rater reliability (i.e., triangulation by researchers).

Context evaluation

The questions in the interview guide for the workers were designed with reference to the CIPP model (9). As far as context evaluation concerned, 11 workers (73.33%) expressed that they had not conducted any systematic drug prevention programs before. Among those who had previously conducted drug prevention programs, analyses of the responses showed that most of the activities were relatively short and unsystematic, such as drug talks, carnivals, and adventured-based counselling camps. The findings are shown in Table 1.

Regarding the mode of evaluation for drug prevention programs held previously, some of the informants had used case analysis and client satisfaction questionnaires. However, 4 workers (26.67%) indicated that they had not conducted any systematic evaluation for such programs. With reference to the question of whether they knew the structured drug prevention programs developed in the West, 8 workers (53.33%) indicated that they did not know, 2 workers (13.33%) said that they had heard of but they did not know much and 3 workers (20%) said that they had consulted local materials only.

Table 1. Workers' responses to the question: "What were the training methods or services provided in the past?"

No.	Content	Responses (N)	Percentage
1	Anti-drug talks	3	20.00%
2	Distribution of anti-drug leaflets	2	13.33%
3	One-shot workshop with games and activities	2	13.33%
4	"Healthy Generation" program	2	13.33%
5	Carnival or exhibition	2	13.33%
6	Participated in a project entitled "Sexual diseases competition"	2	13.33%
7	Alternative activities such as fitness training	1	6.66%
8	Adventure-based counseling or camping	1	6.66%
Total		15	100%

Input evaluation

Regarding the selection of program participants, 12 workers (80%) indicated that the participants were either selected by them in terms of severity of problems or recommended by the school. Only 3 workers (20%) recruited members via open recruitment. Regarding the question whether the workers encountered any difficulties in the recruitment plan, various difficulties were included. In particular, 4 workers mentioned the difficulty of recruiting participants in the experimental and control groups and another 4 workers mentioned the problem of labeling (Table 2).

Regarding the question of whether the implementation of the program had affected the normal work of the workers, 5 workers (33.33%) indicated that the related work was additional and 7 workers (46.67%) thought that the program was part of the normal workload. Concerning the question of whether adequate resources had been planned and arranged, among the 23 responses from the workers, 18 responses (78.26%) were positive. For those responses that were not positive, the problems included difficulty in planning meeting time and inadequate manpower (Table 2). In regard to the cooperation among the school, agency, research team and community, 15 out of the 20 responses were positive. In particular, 4 workers (26.66%) expressed that the arrangement where research team members led the groups was a good arrangement.

Table 2. Workers' responses to the question: "Did you encounter any difficulties in recruiting members?"

No.	Items	Responses (N)	Percentage
1	Difficulty in recruiting members in the control group	4	22.22%
2	Because the school selected students with problems to join the group, some students showed resistance	4	22.22%
3	There were too many sessions and students did not want to use their own time	3	16.66%
4	Attrition in the control group was high	2	11.11%
5	Difficulty in recruiting members because similar programs had been held in the past	1	5.56%
6	Gender ratios were not equal	1	5.56%
7	Objection from the parents because they perceived stigmatizing effect of joining the program	1	5.56%
8	No particular problems encountered	2	11.11%
Total		18	100%

Process evaluation

Regarding the workers' impressions of the program, most of the workers were positive about the program (Table 3) and they felt that there were many positive features of the program (Table 4). In addition, over half of the responses supported the applicability of the program, although the workers also mentioned some obstacles hindering the applicability of the program (Table 5).

Concerning the special experiences of the workers, most of the narrated experiences (12 out of 17 responses) were positive in nature. For responses related to negative experiences, 4 responses were related to the discipline of the members and 1 response was about the members' challenge of the worker. The workers also perceived that the participants were positive about the program. Among the 38 responses, 27 responses were positive (Table 6).

Table 3. Workers' responses to the question: "What is your impression of the program?"

No.	Items	Responses (N)	Percentage
	Positive Responses:		
1	The content was fruitful, systematic, with clear goals	13	38.23%

No.	Items	Responses (N)	Percentage
2	The program manual was helpful to the worker	4	11.77%
3	The content was primarily about drug prevention and related knowledge transmitted through games	4	11.77%
4	The content was related to the themes and rationales of different group sessions	3	8.82%
5	It was helpful to adolescents who had abused drugs	1	2.94%
6	The program evaluation was very systematic and academic	1	2.94%
	Neutral Responses:		
7	The content was rather cognitive	2	5.88%
	Negative Responses:		
8	The content of program manual might not suit the needs of different students	4	11.77%
9	Too many group sessions	1	2.94%
10	Not diverse enough because only group activities were used to transmit the knowledge	1	2.94%
	Total	34	100%

Remarks:
i. Out of 25 randomly selected responses, the first rater and second rater agreed on 20 responses over the categorization in terms of the basic categories (inter-rater reliability = 80%).
ii. Out of 25 randomly selected responses, the first rater and second rater agreed on 22 responses over the classification of positive and negative responses (inter-rater reliability = 88%).

Table 4. Workers' responses to the question: "What are the characteristics of the program?"

No.	Items	Responses (N)	Percentage
	Positive Responses:		
1	The content was mainly about drug prevention and the knowledge was transmitted by games	5	27.77%
2	Wide content coverage with many topics and information was sufficient	4	22.22%
3	A wide range of activities provided	4	22.22%
4	Adoption of a group work approach	2	11.11%
5	The program was coherent, progressive and developmental	1	5.56%
6	The program manual was helpful to the worker	1	5.56%
	Negative Responses:		
7	The messages were too repetitive	1	5.56%
	Total	18	100%

Remarks:
i. Out of 14 randomly selected responses, the first rater and second rater agreed on 11 responses over the categorization in terms of the basic categories (inter-rater reliability = 78.57%).
ii. Out of 14 randomly selected responses, the first rater and second rater agreed on 12 responses over the classification of positive and negative responses (inter-rater reliability = 85.71%).

Table 5. Workers' responses to the question: "What is the applicability of the program?"

No.	Items	Responses (N)	Percentage
	Positive Responses:		
1	Basically appropriate and members were very involved in the group activities	3	16.67%
2	It increased the alertness of the members, especially for those who were curious about drugs	3	16.67%
3	Content was very relevant to the need of schools because many students would come across the drug abuse problems	2	11.10%
4	It could improve family relationship by providing the chance for the parents to join the group activities	1	5.56%
5	The worker-client relationship could be enhanced through the group activities that set the stage for casework	1	5.56%
	Neutral Responses:		
6	It was applicable to docile adolescents but the program needed some changes for those rebellious adolescents	1	5.56%
7	While discussion could be applied to docile members, more activities were needed for those rebellious members	1	5.56%
	Negative Responses:		
8	The content focused on self-reflection, but the members might not be patient enough to think and discuss	2	11.10%
9	It was difficult for the outreaching team to carry out the program because the members from their clientele might not have patience and concentration to participate in all the sessions	2	11.10%
10	Some of the topics in early adolescent group should be amended (especially those about sex) because the content was too difficult for the members	1	5.56%
11	Many "passive" activities were included which were difficult for members to get involved	1	5.56%
	Total	18	100%

Remarks:
i. Out of 15 randomly selected responses, the first rater and second rater agreed on 12 responses over the categorization in terms of the basic categories (inter-rater reliability = 80%).
ii. Out of 15 randomly selected responses, the first rater and second rater agreed on 13 responses over the classification of positive and negative responses (inter-rater reliability = 86.67%).

With reference to the difficulties encountered during implementation, 37 responses were recorded. The informants expressed the following difficulties: cognitive abilities of the members (N=3), discipline problems (N=4), interaction problems among the members (N=5), timing problems (N=7), venue problems (N=1), too many group members (N=2), coordination problems (N=6), manual problems (N=7) and prolonged collection of evaluation data (N=2). Regarding the workers' views on the evaluation of the program, among the 37 responses, 31 responses were negative, such as the lengthy of the questionnaire and it took much time to complete the questionnaire.

Table 6. Workers' responses to the question: "What were the feedbacks of the group members on the program?"

No.	Items	Responses (N)	Percentage
	Positive Responses:		
1	Members were very interested in cigarette and drug because some of them wanted to try and they did not know the harms of abuse	4	10.53%
2	Members were very involved in the group activities and they could grasp the knowledge	4	10.53%
3	Members were willing to share	3	7.90%
4	Members were conscientious	3	7.90%
5	Members learned team spirit	2	5.26%
6	Members were very interested in and willing to share in the two sessions which were about sex	2	5.26%
7	Increased members' consciousness of not taking drugs	2	5.26%
8	Members were more interested in the content which was about pressure, choice and self-image	2	5.26%
9	Members in Astro Kids program enjoyed the group work format	1	2.63%
10	Some of the members were black-listed students and they were very happy to participate in the program because they did not have such chance previously	1	2.63%
11	Group work aroused positive effects on the members	1	2.63%
12	The improvement was very obvious for the Astro Leaders members and they became mature and stable	1	2.63%
13	Members learned to control their emotions	1	2.63%
	Negative Responses:		
14	Members felt bored at the two sessions on drug abuse because the same messages kept repeated	3	7.90%
15	Members felt bored at the topics about cigarette, alcohol and drug because they did not have those problems	3	7.90%
16	Members showed difficulty to grasp the knowledge in reflective activities	2	5.26%
17	The topic about family relationship should involve the parents as well	1	2.63%
18	Members were not involved	1	2.63%
19	The reaction of those who joined in a semi-voluntary manner was not good	1	2.63%
	Total	38	100%

Remarks:
i. Out of 25 randomly selected responses, the first rater and second rater agreed on 19 responses over the classification of category (inter-rater reliability = 76%).
ii. Out of 25 randomly selected responses, the first rater and second rater agreed on 21 responses over the classification of positive and negative responses (inter-rater reliability = 84%).

In short, most of the workers were generally positive about the implementation of the project. They had positive perceptions and experiences about the program and they felt that the members had good responses. They were generally positive about the coordination between the research team and the workers and the related arrangements. However, they expressed concern about the difficulties encountered and the lengthy evaluation mechanism of the project.

Product evaluation

Most of the informants perceived that the project was different from the "conventional" drug prevention programs. A summary of the 20 responses

Table 7. Workers' responses to the question: "Which areas of the group can be improved?"

No.	Items	Responses (N)	Percentage
1	To contain more activities, pictures, and videos because the members were weak at comprehension	4	16.66%
2	To reduce the number of sessions	6	25.00%
3	To improve the concentration of the members, the topics can be broken into more sessions with shorter length of time for each session	3	12.49%
4	The effect of the group can last longer by long-term follow-up work	2	8.32%
5	To delete one session which is about cigarette and alcohol because the members did not have those problems and the problems were also not as serious as drug abuse	1	4.17%
6	To design more challenging activities in order to increase the members' involvement	1	4.17%
7	To provide a list of references and to reduce the content of questionnaire	1	4.17%
8	To rearrange the sequence of the topics by putting the interesting topics at the beginning in order to increase the adolescents' interest to join the program	1	4.17%
9	To improve the member selection method at school; some of the students might be left out if the school only picks those on the list	1	4.17%
10	To explore more about the values of members	1	4.17%
11	To increase the content about family relationship	1	4.17%
12	More continuity and opportunities for adolescents to actualize themselves if they participate at all 3 levels	1	4.17%
13	To involve the teachers so that they can gain the knowledge as well	1	4.17%
	Total	24	100%

Table 8. Workers' responses to the question: "What were the changes of members after joining the program?"

No.	Content	Responses (N)	Percentage
	a. Knowledge, attitude, and behavior related to drugs:		
	Positive Responses:		
1	Increased knowledge about drugs	14	29.78%
2	Attitude towards drug became positive	14	29.78%
3	Increased skills to refuse taking drug	6	12.77%
4	Members abusing drugs had self-reflections. Some of them stopped taking drugs. Some of them reduced the dosage of drugs and frequency of taking drugs.	2	4.26%
5	Some of the members shared what they had learned from the group to those outside the group	2	4.26%
6	Reduced the frequency of going to disco	2	4.26%
7	Reduced smoking	2	4.26%
	Negative Response:		
8	Attitude and behavior changes were not obvious	4	8.50%
9	It was hard to change the values of the members even though they knew their values were wrong	1	2.13%
	Total	47	100%
	b. Knowledge, attitude, and behavior related to sex:		
	Positive Responses:		
1	Increased knowledge about sex	10	50.00%
2	Attitude towards sex became more conservative and conscientious	6	30.00%
3	Learned how to protect themselves	2	10.00%
	Neutral Responses:		
4	Attitude towards sex remained the same	2	10.00%
	Total	20	100%
	c. Other changes:		
	Positive Responses:		
1	Improvement of interpersonal skills	6	20.00%
2	Learned how to respect others and willing to receive advice from others	5	16.67%
3	Increased self-understanding	3	10.00%
4	Increased sense of responsibility	3	10.00%
5	Increased confidence	3	10.00%
6	Became more disciplined and had related changes in behaviors	3	10.00%
7	Improved relationship with teachers	2	6.67%

Table 8. (Continued)

No.	Items	Responses (N)	Percentage
8	Improved emotional control	1	3.33%
9	Learned to express their feelings and opinions	1	3.33%
10	Made progress on school performance and took initiative to study	1	3.33%
	Neutral Responses:		
11	Not much changes in family relationship because some of the members' families did not care about them and others were over-protected by their families	2	6.67%
	Total	30	100%

Remarks:
a. Out of 30 randomly selected responses, the first rater and second rater agreed on 24 responses over the classification of category (inter-rater reliability = 80%). Out of 30 randomly selected responses, the first rater and second rater agreed on 26 responses over the classification of positive and negative responses (inter-rater reliability = 86.67%).
b. Out of 15 randomly selected responses, the first rater and second rater agreed on 13 responses over the classification of category (inter-rater reliability = 86.67%). Out of 15 randomly selected responses, the first rater and second rater agreed on 12 responses over the classification of positive and negative responses (inter-rater reliability = 80%).
c. Out of 20 randomly selected responses, the first rater and second rater agreed on 15 responses over the classification of category (inter-rater reliability = 75%). Out of 20 randomly selected responses, the first rater and second rater agreed on 18 responses over the classification of positive and negative responses (inter-rater reliability = 90%).

showed that the workers perceived the program to be systematic (N=6), rich and continuous (N=3), educational in nature (N=2), cognitive (N=2), long-term (N=2), large-scale (N=1), in-depth (N=1), having aftercare (N=1), adopting group work approach (N=1), and the content might be repetitive (N=1). Generally speaking, the workers perceived that the program was different from the conventional programs in terms of its systematic design and long-term nature. However, some areas for further improvement of the program were also suggested. They are outlined in Table 7.

Regarding the perceived changes in the members after they joined the program, most of the workers expressed that the program had helped the participants to acquire more knowledge on sex and substance abuse and to develop more appropriate attitudes and behaviors in these two domains. The workers were also very positive about the beneficial effects of the programs on the participants. The findings are shown in Table 8.

In addition, 13 workers (86.67%) perceived that the program was helpful to young people in general. However, 2 workers opined that the program might not be helpful for those who were rebellious. The related findings are shown in Table 9.

The perspective of the program implementers

Table 9. Workers' responses to the question: "Do you think the group is helpful for adolescents?"

No.	Items	Responses (N)	Percentage
	Yes:		
1	To a certain extent because it provides an opportunity for adolescents to enrich their knowledge	7	46.66%
2	Helpful with respect to drug prevention	3	20.00%
3	Widens the horizon of the members and provides a chance for them to learn and obey the rules	1	6.67%
4	A source of help for members	1	6.67%
5	Learns correct values	1	6.67%
	No:		
6	Not useful for rebellious adolescents	2	13.33%
	Total	15	100%

Remarks:
Out of 12 randomly selected responses, the first rater and second rater agreed on 10 responses over the classification (inter-rater reliability = 83.33%).

The workers gave 21 responses with respect to the question of why the program was able to bring forth the changes observed. The workers believed that the following factors were conducive to the positive changes in the participants: the use of group discussion and sharing (N=6), information disseminated (N=4), care of the workers (N=4), combination of group and case work (N=2), support provided by the workers and other people (N=2), leadership training (N=1), refusal skills training (N=1) and realization of the members' potentials (N=1).

In addition, the positive effects of the program can be seen in the following narratives of the workers:

Worker 1 (Astro Kids program)

"The improvement was obvious for group members who had progressed from the Kids and Teens programs to the Leaders program. Because of the coherence of the program, they did not only gain more knowledge on drug and sex, but they also became more mature, with positive changes in thinking and behaviors. They could differentiate right and wrong. They also knew that they should not do things such as taking drugs. Besides, members became more self-disciplined and even became leaders. After completion of the Leaders program, members who were rebellious at school in the past changed to be docile and they even guided the others."

Worker 2 (Astro Kids program)

"This program emphasized knowledge acquisition. After playing the games, the worker did not only ask how the members felt, but they also transmitted the correct knowledge to the members. Changes among members could be found during the group discussion. They thought deeply about the messages from the worker. The biggest progress which the members made was they dared to refuse things that they were anxious to refuse in the past."

Worker 3 (Astro Teens program)

"In the past, I thought that drug abuse problems could be intervened by casework only. However, after carrying out this program, I knew that group work was helpful for drug prevention work among adolescents. Also the feedback from the members was positive."

Worker 4 (Astro Teens program)

"Group work is a means for the adolescents to discuss the topics such as drugs, cigarettes, alcohol and sex. Members could express their views and could also influence each other with the assistance of the worker."

The in-depth interview data based on the 15 workers showed that the workers' experiences with the program were very positive. They appreciated the unique characteristics of the program and they felt that the program was different from the conventional programs in drug prevention. They also perceived positive changes in the participants after joining the program and they believed that the program was helpful to adolescents in general. Finally, some areas for improvement and difficulties encountered were revealed from the in-depth interview data.

DISCUSSION

There are several aspects of the evaluation findings based on the workers that deserve our attention. First, the workers were generally positive about the program and they perceived positive changes in the participants after they joined the program. Second, it appeared that it was not common for the workers to carry out systematic evaluation in drug prevention programs and they were not familiar with structured drug prevention programs. Third, most of the workers felt that the evaluation mechanism adopted in the present study was too long and time-consuming.

In their review of the common problems intrinsic to qualitative evaluation studies in the social work literature, Shek, Han, and Tang (6) suggested that 12 principles should be maintained in a qualitative evaluation study. These include: explicit statement of the philosophical base of the study (Principle 1), justifications for the number and nature of the participants of the study (Principle 2), detailed description of the data collection procedures (Principle 3), discussion of the biases and preoccupations of the researchers (Principle 4), description of the steps taken to guard against biases or arguments that biases should and/or could not be eliminated (Principle 5), inclusion of measures of reliability, such as inter-rater reliability and intra-rater reliability (Principle 6), inclusion of measures of triangulation in terms of researchers and data types (Principle 7), inclusion of peer checking and member checking procedures (Principle 8), consciousness of the importance and development of audit trails (Principle 9), consideration of alternative explanations for the observed findings (Principle 10), inclusion of explanations for negative evidence (Principle 11), and clear statement of the limitations of the study (Principle 12). In this qualitative evaluation study, the above principles were upheld as far as possible.

There are three features of the qualitative evaluation findings that make them credible. First, as the perspectives of the workers and the program participants were collected, this can enable us to have triangulation by data sources. Second, quite a substantial number of workers (N=15) and participants (N=30) were recruited to participate in the in-depth interviews. The findings based on the participants can be seen in another paper in this special issue. Although the participants were not randomly selected, the diversity of the informants recruited would generate a fairly comprehensive picture about the informants' perceptions of the program and its effectiveness. Third, inter-rater reliability checking has been carried out, particularly with respect to those questions that are concerned with the benefits of the program and changes in the participants after joining the program. This last feature is a constructive response to the general query that bias may affect the quality of qualitative studies.

According to Shek et al. (13-17), it is imperative to find alternative explanations in the interpretations of qualitative evaluation findings (Principle 10). Fortunately, although there are several alternative explanations of the findings, they can be partially dismissed. First, although the findings can be explained in terms of demand characteristics, this explanation was not likely because the implementers were encouraged to voice out their views freely, and negative voices such as possible areas for improvements were in fact heard. Second, although it can be argued that the favorable findings were due to ideological biases of the researchers, several safeguards (e.g., inter-rater reliability as well as disciplined data analyses and interpretations) were used to reduce biases in the data collection and analysis process.

Nevertheless, the present study suffers from several limitations. First, as the number of implementers that participated in the study is relatively small, it would be interesting if more program implementers joined the research study. It would also be helpful if more implementers stratified according to districts and centre types (e.g., different academic and socio-economical background) could be recruited. However, it is noteworthy that the number of participants is not on the low side. Second, only one-shot interview was conducted for each individual interview, and thus it would be illuminating if regular and on-going qualitative evaluation data could be collected in the group. Third, besides one-shot individual interviews, focus groups and interviews with prolonged engagement would enable the researchers to understand the inner worlds and subjective experiences of the program implementers. Finally, if resources permit, peer checking and member checking should be carried out. Despite the aforementioned limitations, the current study provides additional qualitative evaluation findings that support the positive nature of the Project Astro in Hong Kong.

REFERENCES

[1] Shek DTL. School drug testing: a critical review of the literature. Scientific World Journal 2010;10:356-65.
[2] Narcotics Division. Survey of drug abuse in students in Hong Kong. Hong Kong: Narcotics Division, 2010.
[3] Lam CW, Shek DTL, Ng HY, Yeung KC, Lam DOB. An innovation in drug prevention programs for adolescents: the Hong Kong Astro Project. Int. J. Adolesc. Med. Health 2005;17(4):343-53.
[4] Shek DTL, Ng HY, Lam CW, Lam OB,Yeung KC.A longitudinal evaluation study of a pioneering drug preventionprogram (Project Astro MIND) in Hong Kong. Hong Kong: Beat Drugs Fund and the Hong Kong Youth Institute, 2003.
[5] Patton MQ. Utilization-focused evaluation: The new century text.Thousand Oaks, CA: Sage, 1997.

[6] Shek DTL, Tang V, Han XY. Quality of qualitative evaluation studies in the social work literature: evidence that constitutes a wakeup call. Res. Soc. Work Pract. 2005;15:180-94.
[7] Denzin K, Lincoln YS. The Sage handbook of qualitative research. Thousand Oaks, CA: Sage, 2005.
[8] Stufflebeam DL. The CIPP model for evaluation. In: Stufflebeam DL, Medaus GF, Kellaghan T. eds.Evaluation models: Viewpoints on educational and human services evaluation. Boston, MA: Kluwer, 2000:279-318.
[9] Stufflebeam D, Shinkfeld AJ. Systematic evaluation. Boston, MA: Kluwer-Nijhoff, 1985.
[10] Miles MB, Huberman A. An expanded sourcebook: Qualitative data analysis. Newbury Park, CA: Sage, 1994.
[11] Shek, DTL. Chinese adolescents and their parents' views on a happy family: implications for family therapy. Fam. Ther. 2001;28:73-103.
[12] Shek DTL, Chan, LK. Perceptions of the ideal child in a Chinese context. J.Psychol. 1999;133(3):291-302.
[13] ShekDTL, Lee TY. Qualitative evaluation of the Project P.A.T.H.S.: findings based on focus groups with student participants. Int. J. Adolesc. Med. Health 2008;20(4):449-62.
[14] ShekDTL, Sun, RCF. Qualitative evaluation of the Project P.A.T.H.S. (Secondary 1 Program) based on the perceptions of the program implementers. Int. Public Health J. 2009;1(3):255-65.
[15] Shek DTL, Wong KKL. Qualitative evaluation of the training program of the Project P.A.T.H.S. in Hong Kong.Int. J. Adolesc. Med. Health 2010;22(3):413-23.
[16] Shek DTL, Wong KKL. Subjective outcome evaluation of the training program of the Project P.A.T.H.S. based on qualitative findings. Int. J. Adolesc. Med. Health 2010;22(3):437-47.
[17] Shek DTL, Ma CMS, Sun RCF. Evaluation of a positive youth development program for adolescents with greater psychosocial needs: integrated views of program implementers. Scientific World Journal2010;10:1890-900.

In: Drug Abuse in Hong Kong
Editors: D Shek, R Sun and J Merrick

ISBN: 978-1-61324-491-3
©2012 Nova Science Publishers, Inc.

Chapter 9

EVALUATION OF THE ASTRO PROGRAM USING THE REPERTORY GRID METHOD

Daniel TL Shek[1,a,b,c,d,e] *and Chiu-Wan Lam*[a]

[a]Department of Applied Social Sciences,
The Hong Kong Polytechnic University, Hong Kong, PRC
[b]Public Policy Research Institute,
The Hong Kong Polytechnic University, Hong Kong, PRC
[c]East China Normal University, Shanghai, PRC
[d]Kiang Wu Nursing College of Macau, Macau, PRC
[e]Division of Adolescent Medicine, Department of Pediatrics,
Kentucky Children's Hospital, University of Kentucky,
College of Medicine, Lexington, Kentucky, US

ABSTRACT

The repertory grid method based on personal construct psychology was used to evaluate the effectiveness of the Project Astro in Hong Kong. Thirty participants (N=30) were invited to complete a repertory grid that was based on personal construct theory to provide both quantitative and qualitative data in measuring self-identity changes after joining the program. Both

---

[1]Correspondence: Professor Daniel TL Shek, PhD, FHKPS, BBS, JP, Chair Professor, Department of Applied Social Sciences, The Hong Kong Polytechnic University, Hunghom, Hong Kong. E-mail: daniel.shek@polyu.edu.hk.

quantitative and qualitative data generated from the grid method showed that the participants perceived positive changes in the self-representation system joining the program. This study provides additional support for the effectiveness of Project Astro in the Chinese context. This study also shows that repertory grid method is a useful evaluation method to measure self-identity changes in participants in drug prevention programs.

INTRODUCTION

Because of its high social costs and growing severity in the global context, substance abuse has attracted much research attention from different disciplines. There are at least two challenges faced by the public in the area of substance abuse. The first challenge is related to the change in the meaning of substance abuse. Traditionally, substance abuse closely related to heroin abuse has been seen as a social pathology that should be eradicated. However, with the rise of postmodern thoughts in which the distinction between "right" and "wrong" is rejected, some people start to argue that substance abuse is a "way of life" that does not bring much harm to the addicts. These ideas have much attraction for young people who usually challenge authority figures and views during their adolescent years (1).

The second challenge relates to what effective preventive and treatment approaches could and should be developed. Generally speaking, relapse rates in substance abuse are high while success rates for treatment programs (particularly psychotropic substance abuse) is low. Obviously, there is the challenge to develop effective substance abuse prevention and treatment programs. With reference to this challenge, we definitely need evidence-based prevention and treatment programs. Although there are some successful examples of evidence-based prevention and treatment programs in the West, such programs are almost non-existent in the Asian contexts.

As pointed out by Shek (2,3), evidence-based intervention programs are needed to tackle adolescent developmental challenges. Unfortunately, validated drug prevention program is almost non-existent in Hong Kong. Although many organizations in Hong Kong provide drug prevention programs for young people, such programs often lack vigorous evaluation. In response to this unfortunate situation, Shek et al. (4,5) developed a pioneering drug prevention project in Hong Kong (Project Astro MIND) and evaluated the effectiveness of the related programs. Project Astro MIND comprises three sequential and developmentally appropriate programs (Astro Kids, Astro Teens, and Astro Leaders) designed for children and adolescents, with topics on drug, sex, adolescent development, and life skills with reference to risk and protective factors in adolescent substance abuse, are included in the group sessions.

Several evaluation mechanisms were adopted to evaluate the effectiveness of the Project Astro MIND. First, a longitudinal pretest-posttest control group design was employed to evaluate the effectiveness of the project. For participants in the experimental groups (139 Astro Kids and 217 Astro Teens participants) and the control groups (213 Astro Kids and 201 Astro Teens participants), they were required to respond to objective outcome measures, including measures of social skills, attitude towards drugs, refusal skill towards drugs, usage of drugs, behavioral intention, knowledge about drugs and sex, stress and psychological well-being at pretest and different posttests. Analyses of covariance showed that Astro Kids and Astro Teens programs were effective in increasing the social skills, refusal skills, drug knowledge, and sex knowledge of the participants. Compared with control participants, program participants also had less favorable attitudes towards taking drugs at posttests.

Besides objective outcome evaluation, subjective outcome evaluation based on the perspective of the participants was carried out. Results showed that the participants generally had positive evaluation of the project and they held the view that the project could help them to stay away from drugs. Such findings are further supported by the qualitative evaluation findings based on the participants and workers. The findings based on these two evaluation strategies can be seen in other papers published in this special issue.

In addition to the above evaluation strategies, repertory test based on personal construct psychology was employed to evaluate the Project Astro MIND. The repertory grid test is an assessment method closely related to personal construct psychology that assesses the personal construct system of an individual (6-9).

According to Kelly (8), the universes an ongoing process which can only be understood in terms of construction and re-construction (e.g., from a good marriage to divorce) through the personal constructs which refer to individuals' world views, interpretations and deductions about life. Actually, personal constructs are transparent templates, through which the external reality is understood, or categories of thoughts by which the individual construes or interprets his personal world (e.g., meaningful vs. not meaningful). Personal construct psychology has been used in different areas, including psychotherapy, personality assessment, organizational psychology, and education.

The repertory grid test was designed by Kelly to understand the personal constructs of an individual. In particular, the repertory grid test has been used to understand the self-identity system in numerous studies (10). There are three unique features of the repertory grid test. First, the assessment method assesses the individual's self-identity system from the perspective of the individual (i.e., using the language of the informant). Second, data generated from the assessment method can be analyzed via quantitative as well as qualitative methods. Finally, the repertory grid test is a very flexible method (e.g., adjusting the number of elements and constructs) that can yield very rich information. Borrell, Pryce, and Brenner (11) provided a review on the use of the repertory grid technique in the social work context. Unfortunately, this technique has not been systematically utilized in the Chinese culture in the context of evaluation.

As an illustration, the repertory grid method as an evaluation strategy to examine changes in ex-mental patients joining a holistic psychiatric rehabilitation program was conducted by Luk and Shek (12). The study investigated perceived personal changes in ex-mental patients after attending a psychiatric rehabilitation program in Hong Kong. The program used a self-help group approach with holistic care elements emphasizing physical, psychological, social, and spiritual functioning of the participants. Nineteen participants (N=19) were invited to complete the repertory grid test to measure self-identity changes after joining the program. Ten supplied elements and 10 constructs were elicited from triads. This procedure was intended to produce two contrasting poles for the construct. The constructs were then linked to elements by a six-point rating scale. To assess the self-identity systems of the program participants, the following elements were included: Element 1 (E1: Self Before Joining the Fellowship), Element 2 (E2: Self One Year Prior), Element 3 (E3: Self At Present), Element 4 (E4: Self One Year Later), Element 5 (E5: Ideal Self At Present), Element 6 (E6: My Father), Element 7 (E7: My Mother), Element 8 (E8: One Significant Sibling), Element 9 (E9: An Ideal Ex-mental Patient), Element 10 (E10: An Unsuccessful Person). Regarding Element 9 ("An Ideal Ex-mental Patient"), because every person has some expectations about the "ideal" conditions of a recovering (or recovered) mental patient (e.g., able to work, symptom free, and balanced), this element can be used as the basis to compare the different selves of the participants.

With E5 (Ideal Self at Present) as the anchoring point, the mean distances between E1-E5 and E3-E5 were 1.12 and 0.81, respectively. Analyses showed that the mean distance between E1 and E5 was significantly longer than that between E3 and E5. With the anchoring point on E9 (An Ideal Ex-mental Patient), the mean distances between E1-E9 and E3-E9 were 1.27 and 0.85 respectively. T-test analysis showed that the mean distance between E1 and E9 was significantly longer than that between E3 and E9. When the anchoring point was E10 (An Unsuccessful Person), the mean distances between E1-E10 and E3-E10 were 0.84

and 1.12 respectively. T-test analysis showed that the mean distance between E1 and E10 was significantly shorter than that between E3 and E10. The findings show that all related statistical analyses were statistically significant. It should be noted that the findings were still significant after Bonferroni correction.

In the same study, qualitative analyses were also carried out based on the grid findings. Beyond categorizing the constructs into four domains, the perceived changes of self-representations were analyzed to examine the perceived changes in the constructs by the participants after joining the group. The change in a construct was defined as the perceived difference in a construct between the self before joining the group and the self at present, as indicated by the values of the ratings. The change was positive or negative in the construct-contrast dimension according to the observed scores. The dominant change of a construct is defined as the greatest change of a construct in terms of ratings, when compared with other constructs of the same informant between the self before joining the group and the self at present. Results showed that 18 out of 19 cases experienced positive changes in at least one domain, and some changes were more dominant in certain dimensions according to individual cases. Results showed that while there were perceived changes all four dimensions of the holistic perspective – physical, psychological, social, and spiritual – more changes were demonstrated in psychosocial dimensions. In short, results showed that participants perceived positive changes in physical, psychological, social, and spiritual dimensions after joining the program. This exploratory study suggests the value of adopting a holistic psychiatric rehabilitation approach and provides initial support for the use of the repertory grid method in measuring changes in ex-mental patients in the Chinese context.

Adopting the repertory test methodology, this study attempted to look at how the participants perceived changes in their self-identity system after joining a drug prevention program. The basic expectation was that the program should help the participants identify more with the positive roles, hence protecting them from the negative influence of drugs.

THE REPERTORY GRID TECHNIQUE

This study adopted the repertory grid technique originally devised by Kelly (8, p. 153) in his Role Construct Repertory Test, a method of exploring a personal construct system. A self-identity system put forward by Norris and Makhlouf-Norris (13) was also adopted to measure the self-identification of the clients. By examining how a person would identify himself or herself (self-identification) and the people who are significant to his life, the person's behaviors can be understood. One advantage of the grid method is that it can generate both quantitative and qualitative data in a single study for analysis.

A repertory grid test typically consists of elements and constructs. In the present study, there were 12 constructs elicited from triads. The triads involved selecting groups of three elements from the full list of elements, and the subject was then invited to say in what ways two of the elements were alike and in what way the third element was different from the other two. This procedure was intended to produce two contrasting poles for the construct. The constructs were then linked to elements by a 6-point rating scale. The grid was analyzed by using the INGRID package devised by Slater based on principal components analysis (14).

In the present study, a total of 30 informants completed the grids via a convenience sample. The following twelve elements were used to elicit the constructs:

- Element 1:   Present Self
- Element 2:   Ideal Self
- Element 3:   Future Self (3 Years Later)
- Element 4:   Self Before Joining the Program
- Element 5:   Self After Joining the Program
- Element 6:   Father
- Element 7:   Mother
- Element 8:   Good Friend
- Element 9:   A Drug Addict (Taking Psychotropic Substances)
- Element 10: A Successful Person
- Element 11: An Unsuccessful Person
- Element 12: Form Teacher

The constructs were elicited via the triadic method. For every triad (i.e., three elements in which a self element was presented), the participant was asked to construct in the way that two elements were most alike but were most different from the third one. The participant was generally invited to elicit 12 constructs. After the constructs were elicited, the participant was then asked to rate all the elements on the construct (i.e., along the construct and contrast poles) on a 6-point scale, with 1 to 3 represent the construct pole and 4 to 6 represent the contrast pole.

The raw data for each grid (mostly 12 elements by 12 constructs) were analyzed by the INGRID 72 program (14). In the output of the analysis, there is a section on the distances between pairs of elements. Distances between elements represent for the psychological distances between elements, with a minimum value of 0, a mean of 1 and the value seldom exceeds 2. Therefore, if the distance between a pair of element is close to zero, it means that they are seen as similar in terms of perceived psychological space of the person. On the other hand, if the distance between a pair of element is close to 2, it means that they are seen to be dissimilar in the psychological space of the informant. Norris and Makhlouf-Norris (13) suggested that distances between elements generated by INGRID 72 could be used to examine how a person sees himself or herself as being similar or dissimilar to certain people and others.

To examine the perceived changes of the participants after joining the program, differences in the distances between the following pairs of elements were assessed:

1. The mean distance between "Self Before Joining the Program" (Element 4) and "Ideal Self" (Element 2) versus the mean distance between "Self After Joining the Program" (Element 5) and "Ideal Self" (Element 2): It was expected that if the participants had positive changes after joining the program, the distance between E2 and E5 would be shorter than that between E2 and E4 (i.e., the self after joining the program would be seen as relatively closer to the ideal self).

2. The mean distance between "Self Before Joining the Program" (Element 4) and "A Drug Addict" (Element 9) versus the mean distance between "Self After Joining the Program" (Element 5) and "A Drug Addict" (Element 9): It was expected that if the participants had positive changes after joining the program, the distance between E5 and E9 would be longer than that between E4 and E9 (i.e., the self after joining the program would be seen as relatively farther away from a drug addict).

3. The mean distance between "Self Before Joining the Program" (Element 4) and "A Successful Person" (Element 10) versus the mean distance between "Self After Joining the Program" (Element 5) and "A Successful Person" (Element 10): It was expected that if the participants had positive changes after joining the program, the distance between E5 and E10 would be shorter than that between E4 and E10 (i.e., the self after joining the program would be seen as relatively closer to the successful person).

4. The mean distance between "Self Before Joining the Program" (Element 4) and "An Unsuccessful Person" (Element 11) versus the mean distance between "Self After Joining the Program" (Element 5) and "An Unsuccessful Person" (Element 11): It was expected that if the participants had positive changes after joining the program, the distance between E5 and E11 would be longer than that between E4 and E11 (i.e., the self after joining the program would be seen as relatively farther away from the unsuccessful person).

WHAT DID WE FIND?

Repertory grid test data can be analyzed by both quantitative and qualitative methods (15,16). For quantitative data analyses, many computer programs are available (17). For the present study, INGRID 72 was used to analyze the data, the details of which can be seen in the work of Slater(14). INGRID 72 generates a wide range of information, including distances between elements in the psychological space of the informant. According to Norris and Makhlouf-Norris (13), distance between two elements can be regarded as the degree of similarity or dissimilarity between two elements and this measure can be regarded as an indicator of a person's degree of identification with an element. Stanley (18) used distances between elements to assess psychological and social alienation in young offenders.

GROUP ANALYSES

To examine perceived changes of the participants after joining the program, the distances between the following pairs of elements were compared:

1. The mean distance between "Self Before Joining the Program" (Element 4) and "Ideal Self" (Element 2) versus the mean distance between "Self After Joining the Program" (Element 5) and "Ideal Self" (Element 2).
2. The mean distance between "Self Before Joining the Program" (Element 4) and "A Drug Addict" (Element 9) versus the mean distance between "Self After Joining the Program" (Element 5) and "A Drug Addict" (Element 9).
3. The mean distance between "Self Before Joining the Program" (Element 4) and "A Successful Person" (Element 10) versus the mean distance

between "Self After Joining the Program" (Element 5) and "A Successful Person" (Element 10).
4. The mean distance between "Self Before Joining the Program" (Element 4) and "An Unsuccessful Person" (Element 11) versus the mean distance between "Self After Joining the Program" (Element 5) and "An Unsuccessful Person" (Element 11).

Group analyses of the grid data of the 30 informants showed that the expectations outlined above were supported:

1. The mean distance between Element 4 (Self Before Joining the Program) and Element 2 (Ideal Self) differed significantly from the mean distance between Element 5 (Self After Joining the Program) and Element 2 (Ideal Self): $t=5.32$, $p< .0001$, omega square=0.32. In other words, the informants psychologically identified themselves more with the "Ideal Self" after joining the program. The difference is graphically presented in Figure 1.
2. The mean distance between Element 4 (Self Before Joining the Program) and Element 9 (A Drug Addict) differed significantly from the mean distance between Element 5 (Self After Joining the Program) and Element 9 (A Drug Addict): $t=-4.24$, $p< .0001$, omega square=0.22. In other words, the informants psychologically identified themselves less with "A Drug Addict" after joining the program. The difference is graphically presented in Figure 2.
3. The mean distance between Element 4 (Self Before Joining the Program) and Element 10 (A Successful Person) differed significantly from the mean distance between Element 5 (Self After Joining the Program) and Element 10 (A Successful Person): $t=4.74$, $p< .0001$, omega square=0.26. In other words, the informants psychologically identified themselves more with "A Successful Person" after joining the program. The difference is graphically presented in Figure 3.
4. The mean distance between Element 4 (Self Before Joining the Program) and Element 11 (An Unsuccessful Person) differed significantly from the mean distance between Element 5 (Self After Joining the Program) and Element 11 (An Unsuccessful Person): $t=-3.51$, $p< .0001$, omega square=0.16. In other words, the informants psychologically identified themselves less with "An Unsuccessful Person" after joining the program. The difference is graphically presented in Figure 4.

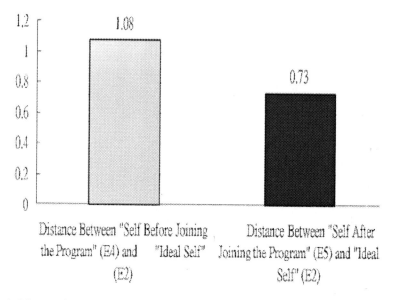

Figure 1. Distance between "Self Before Joining the Program" (E4) and "Ideal Self" (E2) vs. distance between "Self After Joining the Program" (E5) and "Ideal Self" (E2).

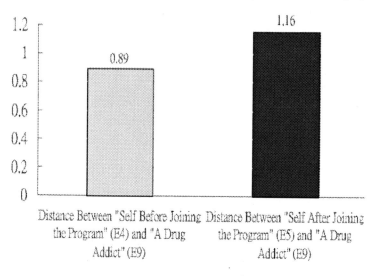

Figure 2. Distance between "Self Before Joining the Program" (E4) and "Drug Addict" (E9) vs. distance between "Self After Joining the Program" (E5) and "Drug Addict" (E9).

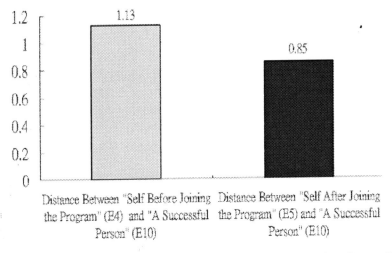

Figure 3. Distance between "Self Before Joining the Program" (E4) and "A Successful Person" (E10) vs. distance between "Self After Joining the Program" (E5) and "A Successful Person" (E10).

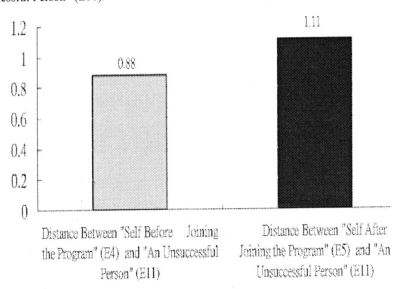

Figure 4. Distance between "Self Before Joining the Program" (E4) and "An Unsuccessful Person" (E11) vs. distance between "Self After Joining the Program" (E5) and "An Unsuccessful Person" (E11).

INDIVIDUAL GRID ANALYSES: EXEMPLAR CASES

In addition to group analyses, data collected by repertory grid tests can also be analyzed at the individual grid level. Two exemplar cases showing drastic positive changes in the informants after joining the program are presented for illustration.

Exemplary case 1 (Informant No. 23)

The informant perceived herself to have the following qualities before joining the program (Element 4): playful, does not understand oneself, has no future, has no goals, failure, non-persuasive, has no self-control, has no power, and does not listen to others (see Table 1).

However, the informant perceived herself to have the following characteristics after joining the program: mature, understands oneself, thinks about the future, has goals, successful, persuasive, has self-control, has power, and accepts others' views.

Table 1. Raw grid data of Informant No. 23

Construct Pole	1	2	3	4	5	6	7	8	9	10	11	12	Contrast Pole
(Mature)	2	1	1	5	2	4	2	2	6	2	5	1	(Playful)
(Understands Me)	3	1	2	5	3	6	3	2	3	2	4	2	(Does Not Understand Me)
(Thinks About Future)	2	1	1	5	2	4	2	2	3	3	4	1	(Not Think About Future)
(Has Goals)	2	1	2	5	3	4	4	2	3	3	4	2	(No Goals)
(Successful)	2	1	2	6	3	3	2	2	5	2	4	1	(Failure)
(Persuasive)	3	1	2	6	2	5	3	3	6	2	5	1	(Not Persuasive)
(No Self-Control)	4	6	5	2	4	4	4	4	1	4	2	5	(Has Self-Control)
(Understands Me)	2	2	2	4	3	6	4	3	5	3	4	2	(Does Not Understand Me)
(No Power)	5	6	5	2	5	3	5	5	2	5	2	6	(Has Power)
(Accept Others' Views)	2	1	2	5	3	6	3	1	6	2	5	3	(Does Not Accept Others' Views)

Elements were used to elicit the constructs

Evaluation of the Astro Program using the Repertory Grid Method   149

Table 2. Changes in the self-identity system of Informants No. 23 and No. 26

A. Informant 23:

Pair of Elements	Distance Between Elements
Self Before Joining the Program (E4) and Ideal Self (E2)	1.888
Self After Joining the Program (E5) and Ideal Self (E2)	0.733
Self Before Joining the Program (E4) and Drug Addict (E9)	0.604
Self After Joining the Program (E5) and Drug Addict (E9)	1.208
Self Before Joining the Program (E4) and A Successful Person (E10)	1.319
Self After Joining the Program (E5) and A Successful Person (E10)	0.293
Self Before Joining the Program (E4) and An Unsuccessful Person (E11)	0.415
Self After Joining the Program (E5) and An Unsuccessful Person (E11)	0.961

B. Informant No. 26:

Pair of Elements	Distance Between Elements
Self Before Joining the Program (E4) and Ideal Self (E2)	1.307
Self After Joining the Program (E5) and Ideal Self (E2)	0.185
Self Before Joining the Program (E4) and Drug Addict (E9)	0.585
Self After Joining the Program (E5) and Drug Addict (E9)	1.558
Self Before Joining the Program (E4) and A Successful Person (E10)	1.307
Self After Joining the Program (E5) and A Successful Person (E10)	0.185
Self Before Joining the Program (E4) and An Unsuccessful Person (E11)	0.585
Self After Joining the Program (E5) and An Unsuccessful Person (E11)	1.558

An examination of the grid data showed that the informant perceived herself to be very close to a drug addict and an unsuccessful person before joining the program. However, she began to identify herself with the ideal self and a successful person but not to identify herself with an unsuccessful person and a drug addict after joining the program. The related findings are presented in Table 2.

The perceptions of the different elements in the psychological space of the informant based on the first factor of the principal components analyses are presented in Figure 5. In the line graph, the findings clearly suggest that the informant perceived that the self before joining the program and the self after joining the program were very different and the positive changes after joining the program were remarkable.

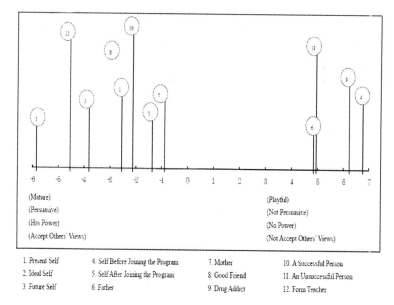

Figure 5. Representation of self and others in the psychological space in terms of the first principal component (Informant No. 23).

Exemplar case 2 (Informant No. 26)

The informant perceived himself to have the following qualities before joining the program (Element 4): not growing, much temper tantrum, dependent on parents, has no self-confidence, has no goals, does not thinking about the future, and active but not serious. However, he perceived he had the following characteristics after joining the program (Element 5): has growth, little temper tantrum, independent, has self-confidence, independent, has goals, think about the future, and silent (Table 3). An examination of the grid data showed that the informant perceived himself to be very close to a drug addict and an unsuccessful person but farther away from the ideal self and a successful person before joining the program. However, he began to identify himself with the ideal self and a successful person but farther away from a unsuccessful person and a drug addict after joining the program. The related findings are presented in Table 2. The perceptions of the different elements in the psychological space of the informant based on the first factor of the principal components analyses are presented in Figure 6. In the line graph, the findings clearly show that the self before joining the program was different from the self after joining the program. The positive changes after the program are obvious and pronounced.

Table 3. Raw grid data of Informant No. 26

Construct Pole	\multicolumn{12}{c}{Elements were used to elicit the constructs}	Contrast Pole
	1	2	3	4	5	6	7	8	9	10	11	12	
(Has Growth)	1	1	1	4	1	1	1	1	6	1	6	4	(Not Growing)
(Communicates)	1	1	2	3	1	1	1	1	6	1	6	6	(Difficult To Communicate)
(Excels)	1	1	1	3	1	1	1	4	6	1	6	6	(Giving Up)
(Little Temper Tantrum)	3	1	1	6	1	1	1	3	6	1	6	6	(Much Temper Tantrum)
(Independent)	1	1	1	6	1	1	1	5	6	1	6	6	(Dependent On Parents)
(Has Self-Confidence)	1	1	1	6	1	1	1	2	6	1	6	5	(No Self-Confidence)
(Motivates To Study)	6	6	6	4	4	6	6	3	1	6	1	6	(Gives Up Study)
(Has Goals)	1	1	1	6	1	1	1	3	6	1	6	1	(No Goals)
(Thinks About Future)	1	1	1	6	1	1	1	1	6	1	6	1	(Does Not Think About Future)
(Studies Well)	1	1	1	3	1	1	1	2	6	1	6	1	(Failure)
(Silent)	1	1	1	6	1	1	1	2	6	1	6	3	(Active But Not Serious)

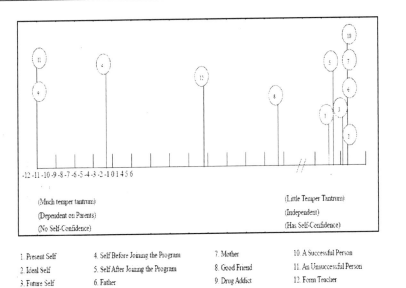

1. Present Self
2. Ideal Self
3. Future Self
4. Self Before Joining the Program
5. Self After Joining the Program
6. Father
7. Mother
8. Good Friend
9. Drug Addict
10. A Successful Person
11. An Unsuccessful Person
12. Form Teacher

Figure 6. Representation of self and others in the psychological space in terms of the first principal component (Informant No. 26).

DISCUSSION

The evaluation findings based on the repertory grid tests clearly revealed the beneficial effects of the Project Astro. Using data based on 30 informants, group analyses showed that the informants identified more with the "ideal self" and "a successful person" but less with "a drug addict" and "an unsuccessful person" after joining the program. Individual analyses using two exemplar cases also illustrated the perceived positive changes in the informants after joining the program. The use of the repertory grid data provides an additional perspective to understand the program effects. Because the repertory grid technique is a 'disguised' form of assessment in which the informants would find it difficult to figure out the purposes of the assessment, the chance of having demand characteristics in the assessment process was not high. As such, the positive findings point to the beneficial effects of the program. In particular, the increased distance between the "present self" and the "drug addict" suggests that the informants are less motivated to take drugs. Because the repertory grid techniques have been rarely used in the evaluation of drug prevention programs, the present attempt is a pioneering effort in the literature. If resources permit, it is recommended that this method should be used to assess the perceived self-identity systems of all program participants.

Borrowing concepts from navigation and military disciplines, Denzin (19) used the term "triangulation" to argue for the utilization of different types of data based on different methodologies to examine the same phenomenon. The basic belief underlying the concept of triangulation is that there are biases in any one type of investigation and such biases and errors would be revealed and cancelled out when different methods, data sources and/or investigators are involved. In other words, triangulation refers to the process of seeking convergence of results based on different methods, researchers, and settings on the same phenomenon under observation. Evaluators generally suggest that triangulation is an important principle that should be utilized to check the quality of evaluation data. When we triangulate the objective outcome evaluation, subjective outcome evaluation, qualitative evaluation, and repertory grid evaluation of the findings in this study, the findings generally suggest that different stakeholders have positive views of the program and there is evidence supporting the effectiveness of the program.

Finally, the present study underscores the utility of using the repertory grid test to assess changes in program participants. According to some researchers, the repertory grid technique can provide data from the informants' own views, and thus represents a better method than questionnaire-type assessments, which may elicit socially desirable responses. With some exceptions, the use of the repertory grid technique is not common in social work field or related professions in Hong Kong. Because of the wide applicability of the repertory grid technique (11), helping professionals should consider using it to assess changes in participants joining drug prevention programs.

Of course, it is noteworthy that there are several limitations of the study. First, the use of convenient sample in the present study casts doubt on the generalizability of the findings. Second, although statistically significant findings were obtained, it should be noted that because of the retrospective nature of the design (i.e., present construction of past roles), the clinical significance of the findings cannot be easily assessed. Third, because there was no comparison group in the study, there is the possibility that the perceived changes in the participants can be attributed to factors other than holistic intervention (e.g., natural maturation changes). Finally, because no manipulation of the independent variable was carried out, the design does not permit us to draw the conclusion that the drug prevention program caused positive changes in the informants. In fact, for those firm believers of positivistic research, they would argue that randomized controlled trial would be the ideal design to examine the issue. While this view is taken, it should equally be noted that experimental approach is not the only approach for evaluation and there are alternative methodological criteria proposed in different paradigms. In addition, it should be noted that there are few studies that utilize the personal construct theory to look at the personal constructions of participants joining drug prevention programs. As such, although the present findings are exploratory in nature, they constitute interesting contribution to the literature.

REFERENCES

[1] Shek DTL. Tackling adolescent substance abuse in Hong Kong: where we should and should not go. Scientific World Journal 2007;7:2021-30.
[2] Shek DTL. School drug testing: a critical review of the literature. Scientific World Journal 2010;10:356-65.
[3] Shek DTL. Enthusiasm-based or evidence-based charities: personal reflections based on the Project P.A.T.H.S. in Hong Kong. Scientific World Journal 2008;8:802-10.
[4] Lam CW, Shek DTL, Ng HY, Yeung KC, Lam DOB. An innovation in drug prevention programs for adolescents: the Hong Kong Astro Project. Int. J. Adol. Med. Health 2005;17(4):343-53.

[5] Shek DTL, Ng HY, Lam CW, Lam OB, Yeung KC. A longitudinal evaluation study of a pioneering drug prevention program(Project Astro MIND) in Hong Kong. Hong Kong: Beat Drugs Fund and the Hong Kong Youth Institute, 2003.
[6] Fransella F. Repertory grid technique. In: Fransella F. ed. Personality: Theory, measurement and research. London: Methuen, 1981:166-77.
[7] Fransella F, Bannister D. A manual for repertory grid technique. London: Academic Press, 1977.
[8] Kelly G. The psychology of personal constructs (Vols. 1-2). New York: Norton, 1955.
[9] Viney LL. Should we use personal construct therapy? A paradigm for outcomes evaluation. Psychotherapy 1998;35:366-80.
[10] Beail N. Repertory grid technique and personal constructs: Applications in clinical and educational settings. London: Croom Helm, 1985.
[11] Borell K, Pryce J, Brenner SO. The repertory grid technique in social work research, practice, and education. Qual. Soc. Work 2003;2(4):477-91.
[12] Luk AL, Shek DTL. Perceived personal changes in Chinese ex-mental patients attending a holistic psychiatric rehabilitation program. Soc. Behav. Pers. 2006;34(8):939-54.
[13] Norris H, Makhlouf-Norris F. The measurement of self-identity. In: Slater P. ed.Explorations of intrapersonal space. Chichester: Wiley, 1976:79-82.
[14] Slater P. The measurement of interpersonal space by grid technique (Vol. 2). Chichester: Wiley, 1977.
[15] Adams-Webber JR. Some reflections on the "meaning" of repertory grid responses. Int. J. Pers. Construct. Psychol. 1989;2:77-92.
[16] Bannister D. The rationale and clinical relevance of repertory grid technique.Br. J.Psychiat.1965;111:977-82.
[17] Shaw MLG. Recent advances in personal construct technology. London: Academic Press, 1981.
[18] Stanley B. Alienation in young offenders. In: Beail N. ed. Repertory grid technique and personal constructs: applications in clinical and educational settings. London: Croom Helm, 1985:47-60.
[19] Denzin NK. The research act: A theoretical introduction to sociological methods. New York: McGraw-Hill, 1978.

In: Drug Abuse in Hong Kong
Editors: D Shek, R Sun and J Merrick
ISBN: 978-1-61324-491-3
©2012 Nova Science Publishers, Inc.

Chapter 10

PREVALENCE AND PSYCHOSOCIAL CORRELATES

Daniel TL Shek[1,a,b,c,d,e] *and Cecilia MS Ma*[a]

[a]Department of Applied Social Sciences,
The Hong Kong Polytechnic University, Hong Kong, PRC
[b]Public Policy Research Institute,
The Hong Kong Polytechnic University, Hong Kong, PRC
[c]East China Normal University, Shanghai, PRC
[d]Kiang Wu Nursing College of Macau, Macau, PRC
[e]Division of Adolescent Medicine, Department of Pediatrics,
Kentucky Children's Hospital, University of Kentucky,
College of Medicine, Lexington, Kentucky, US

ABSTRACT

Smoking, drinking and abuse of illicit drug behavior were examined in 3,328 Secondary 1 students in Hong Kong. Results showed that 5.8% and 28% of the respondents indicated that they had smoked and consumed alcohol in the past year, respectively. Some students had consumed organic solvent (2.1%), cough mixture (0.5%) and ketamine (0.4%) in the past year.

---

[1]Correspondence: Professor Daniel TL Shek, PhD, FHKPS, BBS, JP, Chair Professor, Department of Applied Social Sciences, The Hong Kong Polytechnic University, Hunghom, Hong Kong. E-mail: daniel.shek@polyu.edu.hk.

Results showed that different measures of positive youth development and family functioning were related to adolescent substance abuse behavior. Generally speaking, higher levels of positive youth development and favorable family functioning were related to lower levels of substance abuse. The contribution of positive youth development and family factors to adolescent substance abuse is discussed.

INTRODUCTION

Based on the findings reported in some of the major databases on adolescent development such as Monitoring the Future (MTF), Youth Risk Behavior Surveillance(YRBS) and National Household Survey on Drug Abuse (NHSDA), adolescent substance abuse is a concern for policy makers and health professionals due to the rising of youth substance use (1). For example, from the results of the 2008 National Survey on Drug Use and Health, it was found that 9.3 percent of youths aged 12 to 17 were current illicit drug users (2).

The prevalence of substance use was not only found in North America and European countries, but also in Asian countries. With particular reference to Hong Kong, Shek (3) highlighted the following phenomena in substance abuse trend among adolescents in Hong Kong. First, there were two peaks in the number of substance abusers in the past decade. The first peak was in 1994 where the increase was due to abuse of tranquilizers and depressants. The second peak was in 2000 where the increase was related to the abuse of stimulants such as ecstasy and the rave party culture. Second, regarding the types of drugs abused, statistics show that psychotropic substances (particularly ketamine) were the major choice of abuse in recent years. Consistent with some recent research findings, cough medicine abuse was also rising. Third, regarding the reasons why young people in Hong Kong abuse drugs, peer influence and curiosity are two major reasons why young people abuse drugs. Shek (3) further outlined factors on different ecological levels which contribute to the rising adolescent substance abuse trend in Hong Kong. For example, on the personal level, research findings showed that several factors predispose adolescent substance abuse problem. These include curiosity, material affluence, "green house" upbringing process, lack of life meaning, and few systematic life skills and positive youth development programs in the formal curriculum in Hong Kong. Based on the ecological model, Shek (3) discussed the strategies to cope with adolescent substance abuse in Hong Kong. To date, however, there are no regular surveys of substance abuse among young people in Hong Kong except those school surveys conducted by the Narcotics

Division of the Government of the Hong Kong Special Administrative Region in an irregular basis. Obviously, there is a need to examine the profiles of substance abuse in young people in Hong Kong.

Researchers and practitioners play an important role in helping young people from raising their awareness of the detrimental effect of drugs and developing positive psychological well-being. Effort in addressing the growing profile of drug abuse has been repeatedly emphasized at the national and international levels (4,5). Actually, scholars proposed prevention of substance abuse program should focus on building competence and resilience by adopting the positive youth development (PYD) approach to buffer against the risk of addictive behavior (6-8). In particular, identification of risk and protective factors is an important step in formulating strategies to combat the problem. However, the majority of the substance use studies were conducted in the western countries. Given the upsurge of the nonmedical psychotropic and illicit drug use has become a global public health issue, more research in examining factors that work against youth substance use, especially in the Chinese context, is warranted.

There are two factors that are intimately related to adolescent problem behavior. First, positive youth development constructs are proposed to be related to adolescent problem behavior such as substance abuse. As adolescents having weak resilience, poor psychosocial competencies, blurred self-identity, and low self-efficacy are likely to have poor developmental outcomes, there are theoretical accounts regarding the influence of positive youth development on mitigating adolescent problem behavior. Based on the concepts of protective factors in resilience literature, it can be conjectured that internal resources such as psychosocial competencies and external resources such as bonding (9) would protect individuals from life stresses, thereby minimizing the occurrence of problem behavior. There are researches showing that positive youth development was negatively related to problem behavior, such as substance abuse and delinquency. In North America, Catalano et al. (6) showed that around 96 percent of the 25 well-evaluated positive youth development programs reduced problem behaviour. In Hong Kong, Shek (10) found that positive youth behaviour was negatively related to behavioural intention to engage in problem behaviour among Chinese adolescents. Based on a large sample of Chinese adolescents in Hong Kong, there are research findings showing that positive youth development predicted adolescent problem behaviour via life satisfaction (11).

Second, family processes also play an important role in adolescent problem behavior. There are research findings showing that weak parental monitoring and lack of parental warmth predicted adolescent substance abuse; poor family functioning was also conducive to adolescent problem behavior, including substance abuse(12,13). Furthermore, low parental monitoring and greater amount of time spent in unsupervised peer settings predicted higher risk of exposure to substance use among adolescents (14). In the local context, Shek (15) also showed that poor parenting and family dysfunction predicted adolescent problem behavior.

Unfortunately, a review of the literature shows that there are limited number of studies examining the relationships between positive youth development and family processes and adolescent substance abuse in the Chinese context. Against this background, the primary goals of the study were a) to explore the prevalence of substance use among Hong Kong adolescents, b) to assess the relationships between the positive youth development constructs and family functioning and adolescent substance abuse, and c) to examine the predictive effect of positive youth development and family functioning on substance use utilizing cross-sectional data.

YOUTH DEVELOPMENT PROJECT

The data were derived from the first wave of a six-year longitudinal study in assessing adolescents' development and their families in Hong Kong. A total of 3,328 Secondary 1 students (Grade 7) from 28 schools participated in this study. Among the participants, 1,731 (52%) were boys and 1,597 (48%) were girls. The mean age of the participants was 12.6 years old. The demographic information of the participants is shown in Table 1.

During data collection, the purpose of the study was mentioned and confidentiality of the collected data was repeatedly emphasized to all students in attendance on the day of testing. Parental and student consent had been obtained prior to data collection. All participants responded to all scales in the questionnaire in a self-administration format. Adequate time was provided for the participants to complete the questionnaire. A trained research assistant was present throughout the administration process.

Instruments

The Chinese Positive Youth Development Scale (CPYDS)
The Chinese Positive Youth Development Scale (CPYDS, 16) was to assess positive youth development. The CPYDS has 15 subscales, including bonding

Table 1. Socio-demographic profiles of respondents (N=3,328)

	N	%
Gender		
Male	1,731	52
Female	1,597	48
Place of birth		
Hong Kong	2,596	78
Mainland China	665	20
Others	67	2
School (N=28)		
District		
Hong Kong Island	5	18
Kowloon	7	25
New Territories	16	57
Parents' marital status		
Divorced	233	7
Separated	67	2
First marriage	2,796	84
Second marriage	133	4
Others	99	3
Receiving financial aids		
Yes	2,629	79
No	233	7
Others	466	14

(BO), resilience (RE), social competence (SC), recognition for positive behavior (PB), emotional competence (EC), cognitive competence (CC), behavioral competence (BC), moral competence (MC), self-determination (SD), self-efficacy (SE), clear and positive identity (SI), beliefs in the future (BF), prosocial involvement (PI), prosocial norms (PN), and spirituality (SP). The details of the items can be seen in Shek et al. (16). A 6-point Likert scale (1=strongly disagree to 6=strongly agree) was used to assess the responses of the participants. A composite score was calculated by averaging all item scores in order to obtain the mean of the overall positive youth development (CPYDS).

Using multigroup confirmatory factor analyses (MCFA), Shek and Ma (17) showed that there are 15 basic dimensions of the CPYDS could be subsumed under four higher-order factors, including cognitive-behavioral competencies (CBC), prosocial attributes (PA), positive identity (PID) and general positive youth development qualities (GPYDQ). Evidence of factorial invariance in terms of configuration, first-order factor loadings, second-order factor loadings,

The Chinese Family Assessment Instrument (CFAI)

The Chinese Family Assessment Instrument (CFAI) was used to assess family functioning. In the present study, three subscales, including mutuality (mutual support, love and concern among family members), communication (frequency and nature of interaction among family members), conflicts and harmony (presence of conflicts and harmonious behavior in the family) were examined. The five response options were "very similar," "somewhat similar," "neither similar nor dissimilar," "somewhat dissimilar," and "very dissimilar." A higher total score on the subscales indicated a higher level of positive family functioning. A composite score was calculated by averaging all item scores in order to obtain the mean of the overall family functioning (CFAI). The reliability and validity of the CFAI were supported in previous studies (18-21). Furthermore, multigroup confirmatory factor analyses (MCFA) showed the existence of two higher order factors (i.e., family interaction and parenting) and factorial invariance of the CFAI across gender and subgroups (22).

Substance use

Eight items were used to assess the participants' frequency of using different types of substance (i.e., alcohol, tobacco, ketamine, cannabis, cough mixture, organic solvent, heroin, and pills such as ecstasy and methaqualone) during the last year. Participants answered on a 6-point Likert-scale (0 = never; 1 = 1-2 times; 2 = 3-5 times; 3 = more than 5 times; 4 = several times a month; 5 = several times a week; 6 = daily). A composite score was calculated by averaging all eight item scores in order to obtain the mean of the overall substance use. In addition, separate analyses were carried out by combining "smoking" and "drinking" as an indicator and aggregation of other illicit drugs as another indicator.

Family background

An item was asked to assess whether participants received financial aids (known as CSSA - comprehensive social security assistance) from the government of Hong Kong for financial needs. For example *"Your family is now receiving CSSA?"* (1=Yes; 0=No). Furthermore, participants' parents current marital status was asked (1=divorced; 2=separated; 3=first marriage; 4=second marriage; 5=others).

Table 2. Past year substance use among respondents

	Never	Occasionally 1-2 times (%)	Occasionally 3-5 times (%)	Occasionally More than 5 times (%)	Several times a month (%)	Often Several times a week (%)	Daily (%)
Smoking	94.2	2.9	.9	1.1	.4	.3	.2
Drinking	72.0	14.6	4.9	6.1	1.9	.4	.1
Ketamine	99.6	.2	.1	.1	.0	.0	.0
Cannabis	99.9	.0	.1	.0	.0	.0	.0
Cough mixture	99.5	.3	.0	.2	.0	.0	.0
Organic solvent	97.9	1.4	.1	.4	.1	.1	.0
Pills*	99.9	.0	.0	.0	.1	.0	.0
Heroin	99.9	.0	.0	.0	.0	.0	.1

*Pills: such as ecstasy and methaqualone.

OUR FINDINGS

The prevalence of substance use among Hong Kong adolescentsis shown in Table 2. Among the eight types of substance use, nearly 100% of adolescents reported they had never used psychotropic and illicit drugs over the past year. However, about six percent reported past year cigarette use. In addition, almost 28 percent reported they used alcohol during the past year.

Analyses based on Pearson correlation showed that all positive youth development and family functioning measures were negatively correlated (ranging from -.05 to -.17) with the overall substance use. In general, higher levels of positive youth development and family functioning were related to a lower engagement level of substance use (Table 3). These findings are consistent with the expectations of the study.

To examine the relative contribution of different aspects of positive youth development to adolescent substance use, multiple regression analyses were performed with positive youth development measures as the predictors and different measures of substance use as the criterion variables. The findings based on multiple regression analyses can be seen in Table 4. Results showed that bonding (BO), recognition for positive behavior (PB), emotional competence

Table 3. Correlations among variables in the model

	Overall Substance use
Subscales based on primary-order factors	
BO	-.17
RE	-.11
SC	-.05
PB	-.16
EC	-.13
CC	-.08
BC	-.09
MC	-.14
SD	-.07
SE	-.06
SI	-.06
BF	-.12
PI	-.12
PN	-.19
SP	-.15
Subscales based on second-order factors	
CBC	-.10
PA	-.17
GPYDQ	-.17
PID	-.10
Subscales based on family functioning	
Mutuality	-.16
Harmony	-.14
Communication	-.18

Note. BO: bonding; RE: resilience; SC: social competence; PB: recognition for positive behavior; EC: emotional competence; CC: cognitive competence; BC: behavioral competence; MC: moral competence; SD: self-determination; SE: self-efficacy; SI: clear and positive identity; BF: beliefs in the future; PI: prosocial involvement; PN: prosocial norms; SP: spirituality; CBC: cognitive-behavioral competencies second-order factor; PA: prosocial attributes second-order factor; GPYDQ: general positive youth development qualities second-order factor; PID: positive identity second-order factor.

*All correlations are significant ($p < .01$).

Table 4. Regression analyses based on the positive youth development constructs and family functioning dimensions

Predictor	Overall Substance use R	R^2	β^a	Smoking and Drinking R	R^2	β^a	Other Substance use[#] R	R^2	β^a
Subscales based on primary-order factors									
BO			-.07*			-.09**			
RE									

	SC .11** Overall Substance use			.09** Smoking and Drinking			.07* Other Substance use[#]		
Predictor	R	R^2	β^a	R	R^2	β^a	R	R^2	β^a
PB			-			-			
			.07**			.09**			
EC			-			-			-.08*
			.13**			.13**			
CC			.11**			-.08*			
BC									
MC			-			-			
			.07**			.09**			
SD									
SE									
SI			.13**			.11**			
BF			-.07*			-.08*			
PI			.06*						-.07*
PN			-.11**			-.12**			-.08**
SP			-.09**			-.10**			
Model	.29	.08		.29	.08		.15	.02	
Subscales based on second-order factors									
CBC			.14**			.13**			.09**
PA			-			-			-.08*
			.12**			.10**			
GPYDQ			-			-			-.11**
			.27**			.27**			
PID			.08**			.08*			
Model	.23	.05		.22	.05		.12	.01	
Subscales based on family functioning									
Mutuality									
Harmony			-			-			
			.07**			.10**			
Communication			-			-			
			.11**			.11**			
Model	.19	.04		.20	.04				

Note. BO: bonding; RE: resilience; SC: social competence; PB: recognition for positive behavior; EC: emotional competence; CC: cognitive competence; BC: behavioral competence; MC: moral competence; SD: self-determination; SE: self-efficacy; SI: clear and positive identity; BF: beliefs in the future; PI: prosocial involvement; PN: prosocial norms; SP: spirituality; CBC: cognitive-behavioral competencies second-order factor; PA: prosocial attributes second-order factor; GPYDQ: general positive youth development qualities second-order factor; PID: positive identity second-order factor. # Ketamine, cannabis, cough mixture, organic solvent, pills and heroin.
[a] Standardized coefficients.
*p < .05, **p < .01.

(EC), moral competence (MC), beliefs in the future (BF), prosocial norms (PN), spirituality (SP), general positive youth development qualities second-order factor

(GPYDS)and prosocial attributes second-order factor (PA)negatively predicted overall substance use.

However, it is noteworthy that social competence (SC), cognitive competence (CC), clear and positive identity (SI), cognitive-behavioral second-order factor (CBC) and positive identity second-order factor (PID) positively predicted past year overall substance use.

Additional analyses were carried out to examine the influence of different aspects of family functioning to adolescent substance abuse. Consistent with the results of the positive youth development constructs, all family functioning dimensions, except mutuality, were negatively related to substance use (Table 4). However, these relationships were not shown in predicting illicit drug use. In other words, favorable family functioning was associated with lower likelihood of substance use. Furthermore, respondents whose parents were remarried were likely to have a higher level of overall substance use (Table 5). Overall speaking, both positive youth development and family functioning negatively predicted adolescent substance abuse.

Table 5. Regression analyses based on the positive youth development constructs and family background

Predictor	Substance use		
	R	R^2	β^a
CPYDS			-.10**
CFAI			-.15**
Marital status			
Divorced			
Separated			
First marriage[#]			
Second marriage			.05*
Financial aids			
CSSA^			
Model	.23	.05	

Note. Financial aids (1 = Yes; 0 = No). CPYDS=average mean score of all items from the Chinese Positive Youth Development Scale; CFAI=average mean score of all items from the Chinese Family Assessment Instrument.
^CSSA: comprehensive social security assistance.
[a] Standardized coefficients.
[#] as reference group.

*p < .05.

DISCUSSION

The goal of the current study was to examine the prevalence and psychosocial correlates of substance use among Chinese adolescents in Hong Kong. There are several unique characteristics of the present study. First, in view of the paucity of research in different Chinese contexts, Chinese adolescents were recruited. Second, a large sample size was employed to give a more general picture of the problem. Finally, two validated measures of positive youth development and family functioning in the Chinese contexts were used. This study is a positive response to the scarcity of substance use research in different Chinese contexts. It provides insights into the adolescents' involvement in overall substance use and design of appropriate prevention strategies for Chinese young people.

In the present study, the rates of substance use among Hong Kong adolescents are generally lower than those found in North America (23, 24) and European countries (25). Among the types of substance use, drinking alcohol was the most popular activity, followed by smoking cigarette and use of other drugs is the least popular. These findings are in line with previous studies based on a sample of Hong Kong adolescents with similar demographic background (26-28).

Although the rates of drinking and smoking remain low as compared to the findings in the West, the steady trend in substance use deserves our attention due to the inter-correlated nature of problem behaviors (29, 30). This is further supported by a recent survey based on a sample of Hong Kong primary and secondary students. Lau and Kan (26) found that individuals who smoked and drank were likely to engage in other risk and problem behaviors (e.g., truancy, runaway, gang involvement, sexual activity, gambling), and these associations were particularly strong for smoking. As early onset of substance use is linked to later problem behaviors and chronic drug abuse (31, 32), early identification and prevention of substance use among Hong Kong adolescents is needed.

The findings of this study reinforce the notion that higher level of positive youth development qualities would predict lower level of youth risk behaviors (6, 33). The associations between the positive youth development qualities and substance use support the notion that building adolescents' competencies and providing an atmosphere that emphasizing the negative attitude towards substance use would reduce the abuse of alcohol, tobacco, and other drugs (34).Interestingly, several positive youth development constructs (i.e., social competence, cognitive competence, clear and positive identity, cognitive-behavioral competencies second-order factor, positive identity second-order factor) positively predicted substance use. This might be related to the popularity of recreational drug use among Hong Kong adolescents. Data from the Central Registry of Drug Abuse (CRDA) showed that the change of drug use location from public setting, such as disco and Karaoke (41% in 2007 and 34% in 2008) to private settings, such as friends' home, park and public toilet (60% in 2007 and 68% in 2008) among youths under aged 21 (35). Another possible explanation is that for those who are socially and cognitively more mature may overestimate their abilities and thus are tempted to try substances.

Adolescents have a higher chance for engaging in risk-taking behavior than other age-groups under the influence of peer pressure (36, 37). According to problem behavior theory (38), the likelihood of engaging in health-risky behavior would depend on the exposure of risk and protective factors, such as unhealthy models from the significant others, exposure to risk opportunity, and individuals' personal characteristics. This is supported by Graham et al. (39) who found that *"explicit offers to try alcohol"*, *"social modeling"* and *"overestimation of friends alcohol use"* were significantly related to adolescents' future substance use, regardless of gender. Perhaps adolescents are likely to engage in substance use as a way of seeking identification under the peer influence. More research in this area is needed in the future to better understand the factors associated with Chinese adolescents substance use. It is noteworthy that the predictive effects of these positive youth development qualities on substance were generally low.

One of the uniqueness of the present study is the consideration of factors pertaining to adolescents' family background. The role of family structure and family relations on youth problem behaviors are well established (41-43). In line with previous studies, the likelihood of substance use was higher among adolescents from non-intact families than those from intact families (44, 45). In particular, this study reinforces existing research that negative and hostile family relationships were associated with increased level of individual violence and delinquency (42). This indicates the importance of considering family variables in studying youth substance use.

Despite the above findings, limitations of the present study should be noted. First, as it did not include the influence of peer, it would be interesting to investigate how social process interacts with different positive youth development constructs and its impact on individuals' behavior outcomes. Second, future research in examining the longitudinal effect of the positive youth development qualities on substance use could advance the understanding of the trajectories of adolescents' psychological development and problem behaviors. This is supported by recent longitudinal findings which showed that positive youth development programs such as the Project P.A.T.H.S. can help to promote youth development and reduce their negative behavior among Hong Kong adolescents (46, 47).

The present study can help us design prevention substance use programs among youths. As noted by Lilja et al. (48), "Substance use is increasing in many countries...cultural context variables can be collected to enable a clearer understanding of how the environment influences the effects of a prevention program...so that we are able to 'match' a prevention program to different cultural conditions, dimensions, and their unique 'demands' " (p. 335). Clearly, our findings appear to be a positive response to this request. The present study shed light on developing more effective prevention of substance use program among Hong Kong adolescents.

REFERENCES

[1] Johnston LD, O'Malley PM, Bachman JG, Schulenberg, JE. Monitoring the future national survey results on drug use, 1975-2008. Volume I: Secondary school students (NIH Publication No. 09-7402). Bethesda, MD: National Institute on Drug Abuse, 2009.

[2] Office of Applied Studies, Substance Abuse and Mental Health Services Administration, U.S. Department of Health and Human Services. Results from the 2008national survey on drug use and health: National findings. Assessed 2010 Dec 15. Available at:http://www.oas.samhsa.gov/nsduh/ 2k8nsduh/2k8Results.cfm#2.2.

[3] Shek DTL. Tackling adolescent substance abuse in Hong Kong: where we should go and should not go?Scientific World Journal 2007;7:2021-30.

[4] Gruskin S, Plafker K, Smith-Estelle A. Understanding and responding to youth subtance use: the contribution of a health and human rights framework. Am. J. Pub. Health 2001;91(12):1954-63.

[5] United Nations Office on Drugs and Crimes. Prevention of the recreational and leisureuse of drugs among young people.(2002). Assessed 2010 Dec 15. Available at:http://www.unodc.org/youthnet/youthnet_youth_drugs.html.

[6] Catalano RF, Berglund ML, Ryan J AM, Lonczak HS, Hawkins JD. Positive youth development in the United States: research findings on evaluations of positive youth development programs. Prev. Treat. 2002;5:15.

[7] Rich GJ. The positive psychology of youth and adolescence. J. Youth Adolesc. 2003;32(1):1-3.

[8] Seligman MEP, Csikszentmihalyi M. Positive psychology. Am. Psychol. 2000;55(1):5-14.

[9] Jessor R, Turbin MS, Costa FM, Dong Q, Zhang H, Wang C. Adolescent problem behavior in China and the United States: a cross-national study of psychosocial protective factors. J. Res. Adolesc. 2003;13 (3):329-60.

[10] Shek DTL. Positive youth development and behavioral intention to gamble among Chinese adolescents in Hong Kong. Int. J. Adolesc. Med. Health 2010;21 (1):163-72.

[11] Sun RCF, Shek DTL. Life satisfaction, positive youth development, and problem behaviour among Chinese adolescents in Hong Kong. Soc. Indic. Res. 2010;95:455-74.

[12] Rosenblum A, Magura S, Fong C, Cleland C, Norwood C, Casella D, Truell J, Curry P. Substance use among young adolescents in HIV-affected families: resiliency, peer deviance, and family functioning. Subs. Use Misuse 2005;40 (5):581-603.

[13] Wagner KD, Ritt-Olson A, Chou CP, Pokhrel P, Duan L, Baezconde-Garbanati L, Soto DW, Unger JB. Associations between family structure, family functioning, and substance use among Hispanic/Latino adolescents. Psychol. Addict. Behav. 2010;24(1):98-108.

[14] Chilcoat HD, Anthony JC. Impact of parent monitoring on initiation of drug use through late childhood. J. Am. Acad. Child Adolesc. Psych. 1996;35(1):91-100.

[15] Shek DTL. Family functioning and psychological well-being, school adjustment, and substance abuse in Chinese adolescents: are findings based on multiple studies consistent? In: Shohov SP, ed. Advances in psychology research. New York: Nova Science, 2003:163-84.

[16] Shek DTL, Siu AMH, Lee TY. The Chinese Positive Youth Development Scale: a validation study. Res. Soc. Work Pract. 2007;12(3):380-91.

[17] Shek DTL, Ma CMS. Dimensionality of the Chinese Positive Youth Development Scale: confirmatory factor analyses. Soc. Indic. Res. 2010;98:41-59.

[18] Shek DTL. Assessment of family functioning: the Chinese version of the Family Assessment Device. Res. Soc. Work Prac. 2002;12:502-24.

[19] Shek DTL. Assessment of family functioning Chinese adolescents: the Chinese Family Assessment Instrument. In: Singh NN, Ollen-dick T, Singh AN, eds. International perspectives on child and adolescent mental health. Amsterdam: Elsevier, 2002:297-316.

[20] Siu AMH, Shek DTL. Psychometric properties of the Chinese Family Assessment Instrument in Chinese adolescents in Hong Kong. Adolesc. 2005;40:817-30.

[21] Shek DTL. Family functioning and psychological well-being, school adjustment, and substance abuse in Chinese adolescents: are findings based on multiple studies consistent? In: Shohov SP, eds. Advances in psychology research. New York: Nova Science, 2003:163-84.

[22] Shek DTL, Ma CMS. The Chinese Family Assessment Instrument (C-FAI): hierarchical confirmatory factor analyses and factorial invariance. Res. Soc. Work Pract. 2010;20(1):112-23.

[23] Substance Abuse and Mental Health Services Administration, Office of Applied Studies. The National Household Survey on Drug Abuse Report (NHSDA): comparison of substance use in Australia and the United States.(2003). United States Department of Health and Human Services, Rockville, MD. Assessed 2010 Dec 15. Available at:http://oas.samhsa.gov/2k3/Australia/Australia.cfm.

[24] Substance Abuse and Mental Health Services Administration, Office of Appl ed Studies. Results from the 2007 National Survey on Drug Use and Health: national findings.United States Department of Health and Human Services, Rockville, MD. Assessed 2010 Dec 15. Available at:http://oas.samhsa.gov/nsduh/2k7nsduh/2k7results.cfm.

[25] Sigfusdottir ID, Kristjansson AL, Thorlindsson T, Allegrante JP. Trends in prevalence of substance use among Icelandic adolescents, 1995-2006. Subst. Abuse Treat: Prev. Policy 2008;3:12-20.
[26] Lau M, Kan MY. Prevalence and correlates of problem behaviors among adolesecents in Hong Kong. Asia-Paci J. Pub. Health 2010;22(3):354-64.
[27] Lee A, Tsang CKK. Youth risk behavior in a Chinese population: a territory-wide youth risk behavioral surveillance in Hong Kong. Pub. Health 2003;118:88-95.
[28] Lee A, Tsang CKK, Lee SH, To CY. A YRBS survey of youth risk behaviors at alternative high schools and mainstream high schools in Hong Kong. J. Sch. Health 2001;71(9):443-47.
[29] Jessor S, Jessor R. Problem behavior and psychological development:A longitudinal study of youth. New York: Academic Press, 1977.
[30] Lam TH, Stewart SM, Ho LM. Smoking and high-risk sexual behavior among young adults in Hong Kong. J. Behav. Med. 2001;24(5):503-18.
[31] Jackson C, Henriksen L, Dickinson D, Levine DW. The early use of alcohol and tobacco: its relation to children's competence and parents' behavior. Am. J. Pub Health 1997;87:359-64.
[32] Kaplow JB, Curran PJ, Dodge KA, The Conduct Problems Prevetion Research Group. Child, parent, and peer predictors of early-onset substance use: a multisite longitudinal study. J. Abnorm. Child Psychol. 2002;30(3):199-216.
[33] Gavin LE, Catalano RF, David-Ferdon C, Gloppen KM, Markham CM. A review of positive youth development programs that promote adolescent sexual and reproductive health. J. Adolesc. Health 2010;46:S75-91.
[34] Jessor R, Van Den Bos J, Vanderryn J, Costan FM, Turbin MS. Protective factors in adolescent problem behavior: moderator effects and developmental change. Develop. Psychol. 1995;31:923-33.
[35] Narcotics Division. Central Registryof Drug Abuse: Fifty-eight report (1999-2008). Hong Kong: Narcotics Division, Government Secretariat,Government of Hong Kong Special Administrative Region, 2009.
[36] Dahl RE. Adolescent brain development: a period of vulnerabilities and opportunities. Ann. New York Acad. Sci. 2004;1021:1-22.
[37] Spear LP. The adolescent brain and age-related behavioral manifestations. Neurosci. Biobehav. Rev. 2000;24:417-63.
[38] Jessor R, Donovan JE, Costa FM. Beyond adolescence: Problem behavior and young adult development. New York: Cambridge Univ Press, 1991.
[39] Graham J, Marks G, Hansen W.Social influence processes affecting adolescent substance use. J. Appl. Psych. 1991;16(2):291-98.
[40] Eiden RD, Colder C, Edwards EP, Leonard KE. A longitudinal study of social competence among children of alcoholic and nonalcoholic parents: role of parental psychopathology, parental warmth, and self-regulation. Psychol. Addic. Behav. 2009;23(1):36-46.
[41] Graham N. The influence of predictors on adolescents drug use: an examination of individual effects. Youth Soc. 1996;28(2):215-35.

[42] Henry DB, Tolan PH, Gorman-Smith, D. Longitudinal family and peer group effects on violence and nonviolent delinquency. J. Clin. Child Psychol. 2001;30(1):172-86.
[43] Wells LE, Rankin JH. Families and delinquency: a meta-analysis of the impact of broken homes. Soc. Problems 1991;38(1):71-93.
[44] Barnes GM. Impact of the family in adolescent drinking patterns. In: Collins RL, Leonard K E, Searles JS, eds. Alcohol and the family: Research and clinical perspectives. New York: Guilford, 1990.
[45] Haffmann JP, Johnson RA. A national portrait of family structure and adolescent drug use. J. Marriage Fam. 1998;60:633-45.
[46] Shek DTL, Ma CMS. Impact of the Project P.A.T.H.S. in the junior secondary school years: individual growth curve analyses. Scientific World Journal 2011;11:253-56.
[47] Shek DTL, Yu L. Prevention of adolescent problem behavior: longitudinal impact of the Project P.A.T.H.S. in Hong Kong. Scientific World Journal 2011;11;546-67.
[48] Lilja J, Giota J, Hamilton D, Larsson S. An example of international drug politics: the development and distribution of substance prevention programs directed at adolescents. Subst. Use Misuse 2007;42:317-42.

In: Drug Abuse in Hong Kong
Editors: D Shek, R Sun and J Merrick
ISBN: 978-1-61324-491-3
©2012 Nova Science Publishers, Inc.

Chapter 11

A LONGITUDINAL STUDY OF SUBSTANCE USE IN HONG KONG ADOLESCENTS

Daniel TL Shek[1,a,b,c,d,e] *and Lu Yu*[a]

[a]Department of Applied Social Sciences,
The Hong Kong Polytechnic University, Hong Kong, PRC
[b]Public Policy Research Institute,
The Hong Kong Polytechnic University, Hong Kong, PRC
[c]East China Normal University, Shanghai, PRC
[d]Kiang Wu Nursing College of Macau, Macau, PRC
[e]Division of Adolescent Medicine, Department of Pediatrics,
Kentucky Children's Hospital, University of Kentucky,
College of Medicine, Lexington, Kentucky, US

ABSTRACT

Utilizing longitudinal data collected from secondary school students in Hong Kong (N = 7,975 at Wave 1 and N = 6,962 at Wave 6), the present study examined the prevalence of different substance use behaviors among Hong Kong adolescents and identified several psychosocial correlates of adolescent drug abuse. Results showed that drug use was not uncommon

---

[1]Correspondence: Professor Daniel TL Shek, PhD, FHKPS, BBS, JP, Chair Professor, Department of Applied Social Sciences, The Hong Kong Polytechnic University, Hunghom, Hong Kong. E-mail: daniel.shek@polyu.edu.hk.

amongst adolescents in Hong Kong, with alcohol, tobacco, and organic solvent being the most frequently used substance. Being male and non-intact family status were risk factors for adolescent substance use. Consistent with our expectation, good academic and school performance as well as positive youth development constructs generally decreased the likelihood of using drugs.

INTRODUCTION

In recent years, youth substance abuse gains increasing recognition as not only a health issue but a social problem. According to the National Institute on Drug Abuse, substance use is associated with unintentional injuries, homicide and suicides, which are the leading cause of death among U.S. teenagers (1). It has also been reported that regular use of substance during adolescence increases the likelihood of developing drug addition in adulthood (2). The issue of drug use has also posed a financial constraint on the economy of different countries across the world (3).

With the heightened awareness of the issue worldwide, questions of how severe the problem of adolescent substance abuse is, what factors contribute to the occurrence of this behavior, and what preventive strategies should be taken are being asked more frequently. As Shek (4) claimed, there is an urgent need to develop systematic mechanisms related to early identification and prevention for adolescents with high risk for substance use in the family, school, and community contexts. To this end, methodologically sound research studies on adolescent substance use must be carried out.

For the last several years, the prevalence and trends of substance use among adolescents in different countries have been examined through nationally representative surveys by a few international organizations (e.g., Office on Drugs and Crime of the United Nations, National Institute of Drug Abuse in the United States, and European Monitoring Center for Drugs and Drug addiction). The results generally show that the epidemic of substance use in young people varies across countries. For example, in the United States, the Substance Abuse and Mental Health Services Administration (SAMHSA) recently reported that, between 2008 and 2009, while use of alcohol and tobacco among adolescents remained stable, illicit drug use increased from 9.3% in 2008 to 10% in 2009, indicating that illicit drug use may be increasing (1). However, another study in Iceland based on a large sample of adolescents showed that the prevalence of adolescents' use of different types of substance declined substantially from 1995 to 2006. For example, the percentage of daily smoking decreased from 23% in 1998 to 12% in 2006.

With specific reference to Hong Kong, Shek (4) reviewed the reports (from 1997 to 2006) of the Central Registry of Drug Abuse (CRDA) maintained by the Narcotics Division of the Hong Kong Government and pointed out that there was a growing trend of psychotropic substance abuse problem in Hong Kong. In the recent school survey of substance abuse among students in Hong Kong (5), while the proportions of lifetime alcohol- and tobacco-taking secondary students dropped from 66.5% and 15.6% in 2004/05 to 64.9% and 12.2% in 2008/09, the percentages of psychotropic drug-taking students increased from 3.3% to 4.3%. Moreover, among 112 secondary schools that were selected to participate in the 2008/09 survey, drug-taking students were reported in 111 schools. These figures suggest that the issue of adolescent substance abuse cannot be ignored in the society although the present time may not be the worst for Hong Kong in terms of youth drug abuse.

To prevent adolescent drug abuse, the ecological perspective (6) that focuses on risk and protective factors has commonly been used to guide intervention strategies (4). While protective factors are characteristics that decrease an individual's risk for substance use, risk factors increase the likelihood of using drugs. Many prevention studies have attempted to identify the risk and protective factors for adolescent substance use (7, 8), among which the correlation between gender and substance use is well-documented. Overall, males are more likely to use different types of substance, including tobacco, alcohol, and other illicit drugs than females; they were also found to be more frequently involved in drug use than females (9, 10). For example, in SAMHSA's annual survey, 10.6% of males reported past month illicit drug use, compared to 9.4% of females. Moreover, the percentage of males using illicit drugs significantly increased from 9.5% in 2008 to 10.6% in 2009 while the percentage of female users remained fairly stable (1). In Hong Kong, although drug abuse is also found to be more common in males than in females, two new trends on substance use among females are worrying. First, the proportion of female in the total number of drug abusers increased from 18.1% in 2007 to 20.5% in 2008. Second, reported female drug abusers were generally younger than male drug abusers (5).

Family factors are also important predictors of youth involvement in substance use. In the context of Hong Kong, Shek (4) proposed several main factors on the family level that are most relevant to adolescent substance abuse based on a comprehensive literature review. First, both physical and psychological parental absence in non-intact families may contribute to adolescent drug abuse.

Research findings have shown that adolescents growing up in non-intact families are more likely to take drugs than in intact families (11, 12). Second, family poverty may be a risk factor for adolescent drug use. As adolescents with low family economic status often live in a poor community and have limited resources for personal development, they are more prone to academic underachievement and developing pessimistic values and beliefs about having upward social mobility, which may further lead to substance abuse behaviors.

Positive youth development is another important protective factor for adolescent substance use. A number of studies have evidenced that youth problematic behaviors including substance abuse could be more effectively prevented by promoting positive youth development, such as pro-social behaviors, trusting relationships, positive self-identity, a sense of hope, social competence, academic performance, and resilience (13-16). For example, in the Communities That Care (CTC) program, researchers examined the long-term effects of an intervention that incorporate parental education, teacher training, and social competence training on adolescent health risk behaviors for elementary school students living in high-crime communities. By age 18, students who received the full CTC intervention reported fewer numbers of problem behaviors including substance abuse (17). Besides, good academic and school performance was found to reduce adolescent substance abuse.

In the context of Hong Kong, Shek and researchers from five Universities designed and implemented a large-scale youth enhancement program entitled the Project P.A.T.H.S. (**P**ositive **A**dolescent **T**raining through **H**olistic **S**ocial Programmes), which is perhaps the largest positive youth program in Asia (18, 19). The aims of the program are to promote holistic development among Hong Kong adolescents and to reduce their risk/problem behaviors. To evaluate the effectiveness of the program, comprehensive evaluations have been conducted (20-22). The present study utilizes data collected from a longitudinal study conducted as part of the project. The database consists of six waves of data, with more than 6,000 Hong Kong secondary school students participated in the survey at each wave.

There are two major purposes of the present study. The first is to provide descriptive profiles of different types of substance use among Hong Kong adolescents based on a longitudinal sample of Hong Kong adolescents. Given that existing reports on youth drug abuse in Hong Kong are mostly based on cross-sectional surveys, longitudinal study that monitors the prevalence of adolescent substance use behaviors across years would help to draw a more complete picture about this issue. Second, risk and protective factors for youth substance use in Hong Kong are examined, with particular reference to gender, family factors (including family economic status, family life satisfaction, and parental marital status), positive youth development, and academic and school performance. Based on the above literature review, the following hypotheses are proposed: a) boys would be more likely than girls to report using substance; b) family economic status would be positively related to substance use; family life satisfaction would be adversely related to substance use; adolescents who live in non-intact families would be more likely to take drugs than in intact families; c) different positive youth development attributes would be negatively correlated with substance use; d) perceived academic and school performance would be negatively related to adolescent substance use.

A LONGITUDINAL STUDY IN HONG KONG

As part of the Project P.A.T.H.S., details about the procedures and criteria for recruiting the schools participating in this longitudinal study were described elsewhere (25). To iterate, 48 secondary schools were randomly selected in Year 1 (2006), during which Wave 1 and Wave 2 data were collected from Secondary 1 students. Among the 48 selected schools, one school dropped out after Wave 1 and three schools withdrew after Wave 2. In Year 2 (2007), Wave 3 and 4 data were collected from the same cohort who promoted to Secondary 2 by the time, with one school dropped out after Wave 4. In Year 3 (2008), Wave 5 and Wave 6 data were collected from the same cohort in Secondary 3 at that time. The numbers of schools and participants for each wave of data collection can be seen in Table 1.

At each measurement occasion, the purposes of the study were introduced and confidentiality of the data collected was repeatedly ensured to all participants in attendance on the days of survey. Parental and student consent forms had been

Table 1. Number of collected questionnaires across waves

	Wave 1	Wave 2	Wave 3	Wave 4	Wave 5	Wave 6
N (School)	48	47[a]	44[b]	44	43[c]	43
No. of participants	7,975	7,683	7,151	6,811	6,978	6,962
Male	4,169	4,062	3,707	3,500	3,556	3,591
Female	3,387	3,277	3,014	2,896	3,034	3,059
Not specified	419	344	430	415	388	312

[a] 1 school (n = 207) had withdrawn after Wave 1.
[b] 3 schools (n = 629) had withdrawn after Wave 2.
[c] 1 school (n = 71) had withdrawn after Wave 4.

Table 2. Internal consistency and mean inter-item correlations for academic and school competence and positive youth development indicators

	Wave 1 α	Wave 1 mean[a]	Wave 2 α	Wave 2 mean[a]	Wave 3 α	Wave 3 mean[a]	Wave 4 α	Wave 4 mean[a]	Wave 5 α	Wave 5 mean[a]	Wave 6 α	Wave 6 mean
DRUG	.76	.56	.81	.58	.77	.56	.82	.61	.79	.59	.83	.63
ASC	.70	.44	.72	.46	.72	.46	.73	.47	.73	.47	.74	.48
CBC	.91	.38	.92	.42	.93	.45	.93	.45	.93	.46	.93	.46
PA	.87	.40	.88	.41	.89	.45	.88	.43	.89	.44	.89	.44
PIT	.89	.46	.90	.47	.91	.50	.91	.49	.91	.51	.91	.51
GPYDQ	.95	.32	.95	.33	.96	.37	.96	.37	.96	.39	.96	.38

Note: ASC = Academic and School Competence; CBC = Cognitive Behavioral Competence; PA = Prosocial Attributes; PIT = Positive Identity; GPYDQ = General Positive Youth Development Qualities.
[a] Mean inter-item correlation.
All parameters were significant ($p < .05$).

obtained before data collection. Participants responded to the questionnaires in a self-administration format in classroom settings. Adequate time was provided for the participants to complete the questionnaire. A trained research assistant was present throughout the administration process.

Instruments

Consistent with procedures employed in previous studies, participants were required to respond to a questionnaire that included measures of substance abuse, basic family characteristics (i.e., family economic status, parental marital status, and family life satisfaction), positive youth development, and academic and school performance. The measures in the questionnaire are outlined in the following sections. Internal consistency and mean inter-item correlation of these scales at each wave are reported in Table 2.

Substance abuse scale

Eight items were used to assess the participants' frequency of using different types of substance in the past half a year, including alcohol, tobacco, ketamine, cannabis, cough mixture, organic solvent, pills (including ecstasy and methaqualone), and heroin. Participants rated the occurrence of these behaviors on a six-point Likert scale (0 = never; 1 = 1-2 times; 2 = 3-5 times; 3 = more than 5 times; 4 = several times a month; 5 = several times a week; 6 = everyday). As the prevalence of different drug use behaviors is not the same, each item was used as an indicator. In addition, a composite score was calculated by averaging the eight item scores, which was considered a general indicator of drug use.

Basic family characteristics

Three items were designed to provide information about three basic characteristics of the participants' family. First, students were asked whether their family was currently receiving the Comprehensive Social Security Assistance (CSSA), which was used as an effective indicator of family economic status in previous studies(26), with "1" = "receive CSSA" and "0" = "not receive CSSA". Second, family life satisfaction was measured by asking students to rate the extent to which they perceive their family life as happy (1 = very unhappy, 2 = unhappy, 3 = neutral, 4 = happy, and 5 = very happy). The third item asked the students to indicate the marital status of their parents, including "1" = "divorced and not remarried", "2" = "separate and not remarried", "3" = "couple, first marriage", "4" = "couple, second or above marriage", and "5" = "others". Participants' scores on each item were used to reflect their family economic status, family life satisfaction, and parental marital status, respectively.

Chinese Positive Youth Development Scale (CPYDS)

The CPYDS consists of 15 subscales which are listed as follows:

1. Bonding Subscale (six items)
2. Resilience Subscale (six items)
3. Social Competence Subscale (seven items)
4. Emotional Competence Subscale (six items)
5. Cognitive Competence Subscale (six items)
6. Behavioral Competence Subscale (modified five items)
7. Moral Competence Subscale (six items)
8. Self-Determination Subscale (five items)
9. Self-Efficacy Subscale (modified two items)
10. Beliefs in the Future Subscale (modified three items)
11. Clear and Positive Identity Subscale (seven items)
12. Spirituality Subscale (seven items)
13. Prosocial Involvement Subscale (five items)
14. Prosocial Norms Subscale (five items)
15. Recognition for Positive Behavior Subscale (four items)

Based on factor analyses, Shek and colleague (27) proposed that the 15 subscales in the CPYDS could be further reduced to four dimensions:

- Cognitive Behavioral Competence (CBC): Scale score is calculated by averaging scores on Cognitive Competence Subscale, Self-Determination Subscale, and Behavioral Competence Subscale.
- Prosocial Attributes (PA): Scale score equals to the mean score of Prosocial Involvement Subscale and Prosocial Norms Subscale.
- Positive Identity (PIT): Scale score is computed by averaging scores of Beliefs in the Future Subscale and Clear and Positive Identity Subscale.
- General Positive Youth Development Qualities (GPYDQ): Scale score equals to the mean score of Resilience Subscale, Social Competence Subscale, Self-Efficacy Subscale, Moral Competence Subscale, Bonding Subscale, Recognition for Positive Behavior Subscale, Spirituality Subscale, and Emotional Competence Subscale.

These four composite indicators were used to assess participants' positive youth development in the present study. Internal consistency and mean inter-item correlation for each indicator at different waves are shown in Table 2. It should be noted that although the administered questionnaire includes other subscales of the CPYDQ, findings regarding the overall score of CPYDQ and its subscales were reported elsewhere (27). The present paper only focused on the predictive effects of the four second-order positive youth development constructs on adolescent drug abuse.

Academic and school competence scale

As a relatively independent positive youth development construct, participants' academic and school competence (ASC) were measured by three items. For the first item, participants were required to rate their perceived academic performance as compared to other peer students on a five-point Likert scale, with "1" = "very poor", "2" = "below average", "3" = "average", "4" = "above average", and "5" = "very good". The second item asked the extent to which the respondents were satisfied with their academic performance (1 = very dissatisfied, 2 = dissatisfied, 3 = neutral, 4 = satisfied, and 5 = very satisfied). The last question asked the participants to rate their conduct in school on a five-point Likert scale (1 = very poor, 2 = below average, 3 = average, 4 = above average, and 5 = very good). The ASC scale score is calculated by averaging the item scores and ranges from 1 to 5, with high scores representing for high academic and school competence.

Data analytic plan

The first purpose of the present study was to provide descriptive profiles of different types of substance use behaviors among adolescents across six waves of data collection. Therefore, numbers and percentages of adolescents who use a specific type of drug at different frequencies were first computed at each wave. To further show the proportion of participants who reported using substances at least once in the past half year, the percentages of non-zero values on each substance use item were also calculated.

Second, to investigate whether gender, family factors, and positive youth development are predictive of adolescent substance use behaviors, a series of logistic regression analyses were conducted both cross-sectionally and longitudinally, with the composite score of drug use as the dependent variable. It should be noted that although the relationship between age and substance use was not a major focus of the present study, age was also included as an independent variable throughout the analyses to control for its possible effects. In this study, the cross-sectional relationships between different predictors and substance use behaviors were examined at Wave 1 and Wave 6. Longitudinal relationships were investigated by using participants' characteristics at Wave 1 to predict their substance use behaviors at Wave 6.

Specifically, to examine the cross-sectional correlates of adolescent substance abuse behavior, demographic factors (age and gender) were entered in the first block; family characteristics, including family economic status, parental marital status, and family life satisfaction, were entered into the second block; youth development constructs including academic and school competence (ASC), cognitive behavioral competence (CBC), prosocial attributes (PA), positive identity (PIT), and general positive youth development qualities (GPYDQ) were entered into the third block of the regression model. Such analyses were performed twice (at Wave 1 and Wave 6). For the longitudinal relationship, similar logistic regression analyses were conducted, except that 1) the independent variables were data collected at Wave 1 and for the dependent variables (i.e., drug use behaviors) Wave 6 data were used; 2) the composite score of drug abuse at Wave 1 was entered in the first block to control for the effects of initial status of substance abuse in the participants' later drug abuse behaviors.

There are mainly two reasons that logistic regression analyses, instead of general multiple regression, were employed in the present study. First, substance abuse behavior is not a normally distributed phenomenon, and thus cannot be directly used as dependent variable in general multiple regression analysis.

Second, based on a normal youth population, the research interest of this study focuses more on what factors may contribute to whether an adolescent take drug or not than on the relationships between different predictors and the severity of drug abuse behaviors. As such, the composite score of drug abuse was recoded as a dichotomous variable with "0" representing for "never used any type of substance in the past half year" and "1" for "used at least one type of substance listed for at least once to twice in the past half year". In addition, because the variable of parental marital status was categorical in nature, four dummy variables were created: P1 (1 = divorced and not married; 0 = couple, first marriage"), P2 (1 = separate and not remarried; 0 = couple, first marriage), P3 (1 = remarried; 0 = couple, first marriage), and P4 (1 = other situations; 0 = couple, first marriage). The four dummy variables were entered at the second block of the equation.

OUR FINDINGS

In this part, descriptive profile of different types of drug use at each wave is presented first, followed by the results of logistic regression regarding cross-sectional relationships between different predictors and adolescent drug use behaviors. Finally, predictive effects of demographic characteristics, family factors, positive youth development constructs, and perceived academic and school competence of the participants at Wave 1 on their substance use behaviors at Wave 6 are reported.

Descriptive profiles

As mentioned, numbers and percentages of participants who used a specific drug at different frequencies were calculated for each wave of data collection. The results are shown in Tables 3 to 10.

Several observations can be highlighted from the descriptive statistics. First, substance use behaviors were not rare among Hong Kong adolescents across six waves of data collection. For example, at Wave 2, 4% of the participants reported that they used organic solvent at least once to twice in the past half year; 1% of the participants at Wave 6 indicated that they took pills (ecstasy or methaqualone) in the latest six months. Second, alcohol was the most frequently used substance, followed by tobacco and organic solvent, with heroin being the least frequently used drug. Third, while most participants who reported smoking or drinking were

Table 3. Numbers and percentages of adolescents who smoke at different frequencies

	1	2	3	4	5	6	Total Non-Zero
Wave 1 (N = 7906)	283 (3.6%)	79 (1.0%)	77 (1.0%)	25 (0.3%)	30 (0.4%)	56 (0.7%)	550 (7.0%)
Wave 2 (N = 7602)	385 (5.1%)	107 (1.4%)	142 (1.9%)	47 (0.6%)	70 (0.9%)	111 (1.5%)	862 (11.3%)
Wave 3 (N = 7107)	359 (5.1%)	121 (1.7%)	157 (2.2%)	51 (0.7%)	65 (0.9%)	98 (1.4%)	851 (12.0%)
Wave 4 (N = 6749)	397 (5.9%)	119 (1.8%)	148 (2.2%)	63 (0.9%)	90 (1.3%)	142 (2.1%)	959 (14.2%)
Wave 5 (N = 6940)	345 (5.0%)	96 (1.4%)	176 (2.5%)	56 (0.8%)	77 (1.1%)	170 (2.4%)	920 (13.3%)
Wave 6 (N = 6833)	370 (5.4%)	107 (1.6%)	180 (2.6%)	80 (1.2%)	98 (1.4%)	193 (2.8%)	1028 (15.0%)

Note: 0 = never; 1 = once to twice in the past half year; 2 = 3 to 5 times in the past half year; 3 = more than 5 times in the past half year; 4 = several times per month; 5 = several times per week; 6 = everyday; "Non-Zero" means at least once in the past half year.

Table 4. Numbers and percentages of adolescents who drink alcohol at different frequencies

	1	2	3	4	5	6	Total Non-Zero
Wave 1 (N =7887)	1090 (13.8%)	356 (4.5%)	330 (4.2%)	128 (1.6%)	41 (0.5%)	21 (0.3%)	1966 (24.9%)
Wave 2 (N =7577)	1241 (16.4%)	458 (6.0%)	527 (7.0%)	213 (2.8%)	92 (1.2%)	41 (0.5%)	2572 (33.9%)
Wave 3 (N =7075)	1095 (15.5%)	436 (6.2%)	548 (7.7%)	247 (3.5%)	84 (1.2%)	38 (0.5%)	2448 (34.6%)
Wave 4 (N =6743)	1206 (17.9%)	515 (7.6%)	594 (8.8%)	298 (4.4%)	83 (1.2%)	54 (0.8%)	2750 (40.7%)
Wave 5 (N =6913)	1176 (17.0%)	509 (7.4%)	639 (9.2%)	323 (4.7%)	94 (1.4%)	60 (0.9%)	2801 (40.6%)
Wave 6 (N =6846)	1195 (17.5%)	555 (8.1%)	724 (10.6%)	372 (5.4%)	78 (1.1%)	60 (0.9%)	2984 (43.6%)

Note: 0 = never; 1 = once to twice in the past half year; 2 = 3 to 5 times in the past half year; 3 = more than 5 times in the past half year; 4 = several time per month; 5 = several times per week; 6 = everyday; "Non-Zero" means at least once in the past half year.

Table 5. Numbers and percentages of adolescents who use ketamine at different frequencies

	1	2	3	4	5	6	Total Non-Zero
Wave 1 (N =7912)	20 (0.3%)	10 (0.1%)	4 (0.1%)	2 (0%)	1 (0%)	8 (0.1%)	45 (0.6%)
Wave 2 (N =7617)	24 (0.3%)	7 (0.1%)	15 (0.2%)	8 (0.1%)	3 (0%)	27 (0.4%)	84 (1.1%)
Wave 3 (N =7118)	23 (0.3%)	8 (0.1%)	16 (0.2%)	3 (0%)	4 (0.1%)	17 (0.2%)	71 (0.9%)
Wave 4 (N =6774)	24 (0.4%)	8 (0.1%)	14 (0.2%)	9 (0.1%)	4 (0.1%)	31 (0.5%)	90 (1.4%)
Wave 5 (N =6946)	32 (0.5%)	11 (0.2%)	11 (0.2%)	17 (0.2%)	3 (0%)	26 (0.4%)	100 (1.5%)
Wave 6 (N =6813)	32 (0.5%)	8 (0.1%)	26 (0.4%)	12 (0.2%)	3 (0%)	35 (0.5%)	116 (1.7%)

Note: 0 = never; 1 = once to twice in the past half year; 2 = 3 to 5 times in the past half year; 3 = more than 5 times in the past half year; 4 = several times per month; 5 = several times per week; 6 = everyday; "Non-Zero" means at least once in the past half year.

Table 6. Numbers and percentages of adolescents who use cannabis at different frequencies

	1	2	3	4	5	6	Total Non-Zero
Wave 1 (N =7903)	8 (0.1%)	2 (0%)	11 (0.1%)	2 (0%)	1 (0%)	10 (0.1%)	34 (0.3%)
Wave 2 (N =7599)	17 (0.2%)	5 (0.1%)	15 (0.2%)	1 (0%)	1 (0%)	28 (0.4%)	67 (0.9%)
Wave 3 (N =7119)	9 (0.1%)	6 (0.1%)	7 (0.1%)	1 (0%)	3 (0%)	17 (0.2%)	43 (0.5%)
Wave 4 (N =6774)	17 (0.3%)	2 (0%)	12 (0.2%)	1 (0%)	0 (0%)	34 (0.5%)	66 (1%)
Wave 5 (N =6943)	18 (0.3%)	5 (0.1%)	4 (0.1%)	3 (0%)	3 (0%)	26 (0.4%)	59 (0.9%)
Wave 6 (N =6812)	22 (0.2%)	5 (0.1%)	13 (0.2%)	5 (0.1%)	3 (0%)	36 (0.5%)	84 (1.1%)

Note: 0 = never; 1 = once to twice in the past half year; 2 = 3 to 5 times in the past half year; 3 = more than 5 times in the past half year; 4 = several times per month; 5 = several times per week; 6 = everyday; "Non-Zero" means at least once in the past half year.

Table 7. Numbers and percentages of adolescents who use cough medicine at different frequencies

	1	2	3	4	5	6	Total Non-Zero
Wave 1 (N =7800)	40 (0.5%)	15 (0.2%)	20 (0.3%)	4 (0.1%)	3 (0%)	10 (0.1%)	92 (1.2%)
Wave 2 (N =7614)	63 (0.8%)	17 (0.2%)	15 (0.2%)	4 (0.1%)	2 (0%)	6 (0.4%)	107 (1.7%)
Wave 3 (N =7118)	38 (0.5%)	20 (0.3%)	10 (0.1%)	7 (0.1%)	2 (0%)	17 (0.2%)	94 (1.2%)
Wave 4 (N =6774)	41 (0.6%)	11 (0.2%)	10 (0.1%)	4 (0.1%)	1 (0%)	31 (0.5%)	98 (1.5%)
Wave 5 (N =6951)	24 (0.3%)	11 (0.2%)	12 (0.2%)	3 (0%)	4 (0.1%)	25 (0.4%)	79 (1.2%)
Wave 6 (N =6819)	33 (0.5%)	9 (0.1%)	12 (0.2%)	6 (0.1%)	3 (0%)	34 (0.5%)	97 (1.4%)

Note: 0 = never; 1 = once to twice in the past half year; 2 = 3 to 5 times in the past half year; 3 = more than 5 times in the past half year; 4 = several times per month; 5 = several times per week; 6 = everyday; "Non-Zero" means at least once in the past half year.

Table 8. Numbers and percentages of adolescents who use solvent at different frequencies

	1	2	3	4	5	6	Total Non-Zero
Wave 1 (N =7790)	104 (1.3%)	22 (0.3%)	18 (0.2%)	6 (0.1%)	3 (0%)	11 (0.1%)	164 (2%)
Wave 2 (N =7614)	191 (2.5%)	44 (0.6%)	25 (0.3%)	6 (0.1%)	5 (0.1%)	29 (0.4%)	300 (4%)
Wave 3 (N =7118)	114 (1.6%)	34 (0.5%)	29 (0.4%)	7 (0.1%)	4 (0.1%)	16 (0.2%)	204 (2.9%)
Wave 4 (N =6769)	110 (1.6%)	26 (0.4%)	31 (0.5%)	3 (0%)	6 (0.1%)	31 (0.5%)	207 (3.1%)
Wave 5 (N =6945)	89 (1.3%)	21 (0.3%)	29 (0.4%)	7 (0.1%)	3 (0%)	26 (0.4%)	175 (2.5%)
Wave 6 (N =6814)	97 (1.4%)	17 (0.2%)	25 (0.4%)	6 (0.1%)	2 (0%)	35 (0.5%)	182 (2.6%)

Note: 0 = never; 1 = once to twice in the past half year; 2 = 3 to 5 times in the past half year; 3 = more than 5 times in the past half year; 4 = several times per month; 5 = several times per week; 6 = everyday; "Non-Zero" means at least once in the past half year.

Table 9. Numbers and percentages of adolescents who take pills (ecstasy or methaqualone) at different frequencies

	1	2	3	4	5	6	Total Non-Zero
Wave 1 (N =7810)	13 (0.2%)	3 (0%)	5 (0.1%)	3 (0%)	3 (0%)	11 (0.1%)	38 (0.4%)
Wave 2 (N =7620)	13 (0.2%)	5 (0.1%)	7 (0.1%)	6 (0.1%)	2 (0%)	27 (0.4%)	60 (0.9%)
Wave 3 (N =7125)	11 (0.2%)	7 (0.1%)	8 (0.1%)	3 (0%)	4 (0.1%)	18 (0.3%)	51 (0.8%)
Wave 4 (N =6769)	16 (0.2%)	2 (0%)	7 (0.1%)	3 (0%)	4 (0.1%)	33 (0.5%)	65 (0.9%)
Wave 5 (N =6954)	18 (0.3%)	6 (0.1%)	9 (0.1%)	6 (0.1%)	4 (0.1%)	27 (0.4%)	70 (1.1%)
Wave 6 (N =6817)	17 (0.2%)	2 (0%)	17 (0.2%)	8 (0.1%)	3 (0%)	33 (0.5%)	80 (1.0%)

Note: 0 = never; 1 = once to twice in the past half year; 2 = 3 to 5 times in the past half year; 3 = more than 5 times in the past half year; 4 = several times per month; 5 = several times per week; 6 = everyday; "Non-Zero" means at least once in the past half year.

Table 10. Numbers and percentages of adolescents who use heroin at different frequencies

	1	2	3	4	5	6	Total Non-Zero
Wave 1 (N =7801)	6 (0.1%)	1 (0%)	4 (0.1%)	0 (0%)	3 (0%)	10 (0.1%)	24 (0.3%)
Wave 2 (N =7585)	4 (0.1%)	1 (0%)	2 (0%)	0 (0%)	2 (0%)	25 (0.3%)	34 (0.4%)
Wave 3 (N =7124)	2 (0%)	1 (0%)	4 (0.1%)	1 (0%)	2 (0%)	17 (0.3%)	27 (0.4%)
Wave 4 (N =6760)	5 (0.1%)	0 (0%)	2 (0%)	2 (0%)	2 (0%)	32 (0.5%)	43 (0.6%)
Wave 5 (N =6940)	3 (0%)	4 (0.1%)	2 (0%)	2 (0%)	2 (0%)	26 (0.4%)	39 (0.5%)
Wave 6 (N =6813)	9 (0.1%)	2 (0%)	8 (0.1%)	5 (0.1%)	1 (0%)	34 (0.5%)	59 (0.8%)

Note: 0 = never; 1 = once to twice in the past half year; 2 = 3 to 5 times in the past half year; 3 = more than 5 times in the past half year; 4 = several times per month; 5 = several times per week; 6 = everyday; "Non-Zero" means at least once in the past half year.

occasional users (once to twice in the past half year), a large proportion of adolescents who reported taking psychotropic drugs (such as ketamine, cannabis, and ecstasy) and heroin were frequent users. For example, at Wave 6, 33 out of 80 (41.25%) adolescents who reported ecstasy use behaviors expressed that they took pills everyday in the past half year.

Table 11. Descriptive statistics of examined variables at Wave 1 and Wave 6

		Wave 1	Wave 6
Age[a]		3.26 ± 0.94	6.02 ± 1.08
Gender	Male	4169 (52.3%)	3591 (51.6%)
	Female	3387 (42.5%)	3059 (43.9%)
	Unspecified	419 (5.3%)	312 (4.5%)
FES	CSSA	2937 (36.8%)	2767 (39.7%)
	No CSSA	4548 (57.0%)	3759 (54.0%)
	Unspecified	490 (6.1%)	436 (6.3%)
PMS	Divorced but not remarried	532 (6.7%)	575 (8.3%)
	Separate	247 (3.1%)	179 (2.6%)
	Divorced and remarried	256 (3.2%)	309 (4.4%)
	Other situation	288 (3.6%)	252 (3.6%)
	First marriage	6028 (75.6%)	5474 (78.6%)
	Unspecified	624 (7.8%)	173 (2.5%)
FLS		3.75 ± 1.02	3.60 ± 0.96
ASC		3.23 ± 0.71	3.01 ± 0.75
CBC		4.64 ± 0.70	4.61 ± 0.68
PA		4.61 ± 0.80	4.51 ± 0.76
PIT		4.32 ± 0.92	4.27 ± 0.89
GPYDQ		4.62 ± 0.68	4.56 ± 0.67
DRUG		0.10 ± 0.31	0.23 ± 0.58
	Zero values	5791 (72.6%)	3747 (53.8%)
	Non-zero values	2147 (26.9%)	3133 (45.0%)
	Missing value	37 (0.5%)	82 (1.2%)

Note: FES = Family Economic Status; PMS = Parental Marital Status; FLS = Family Life Satisfaction; ASC = Academic and School Competence; CBC = Cognitive Behavioral Competence; PA = Prosocial Attributes; PIT = Positive Identity; GPYDQ = General Positive Youth Development Qualities; DRUG = Composite score of substance use.

For continuous variables (Age, FLS, ASC, CBC, PA, PIT, GPYDQ), values in the cells are means and standard deviations; for categorical variables (Gender, FES, PMS), values in the cells are numbers and percentages of participants. For the variable "DRUG", means and standard deviation based on the original score (continuous variable) are reported first, and then the percentages and numbers of zero versus non-zero values based on the recoded categorical variable are presented.

[a] The reported means and standard deviations for "Age" were based on its original coding where "1" = "10 years old or below"; "2" = "11 years old"; "3" = "12 years old"; "4" = "13 years old"; "5" = "14 years old"; "6" = "15 years old"; "7" = "16 years old"; "8" = "17 years old"; "9" = "18 years old"; "10" = "19 years old"; "11" = "20 years old or above".

Table 12. Pearson's correlation coefficients among continuous variables at Wave 1 and Wave 6

	Age	FLS	ASC	CBC	PA	PIT	GPYDQ	DRUG	Wave1 <--> Wave 6
Age K1	--	-0.13**	-0.12**	-0.05**	-0.09**	-0.08**	-0.07**	0.19**	0.01
FLS K8	-0.06**	--	0.36**	0.39**	0.37**	0.42**	0.51**	-0.15**	-0.08**
ASC	-0.01	0.32**	--	0.41**	0.36**	0.55**	0.45**	-0.09**	-0.10**
CBC	0.01	0.34**	0.31**	--	0.69**	0.72**	0.84**	-0.14**	-0.10**
PA	0.02	0.33**	0.28**	0.65**	--	0.63**	0.75**	-0.18**	-0.10**
PIT	-0.01	0.38**	0.49**	0.74**	0.60**	--	0.75**	-0.12**	-0.07**
GPYDQ	0.03*	0.47**	0.39**	0.84**	0.73**	0.77**	--	-0.19**	-0.12**
DRUG	0.08**	-0.11	-0.03*	-0.12**	-0.14**	-0.09**	-0.15**	--	0.19**

Notes: FES = Family Economic Status; FLS = Family Life Satisfaction; ASC = Academic and School Competence; CBC = Cognitive Behavioral Competence; PA = Prosocial Attributes; PIT = Positive Identity; GPYDQ = General Positive Youth Development Qualities; DRUG = Composite score of substance use.

Values above the diagonal are correlation coefficients at Wave 1; values below the diagonal are correlation coefficients for Wave 6.

Values in the last column represent for the correlation coefficient between Wave 1 predictors (i.e., Age, FLS, ASC, CBC, PA, PIT, GPYDQ, and DRUG at Wave 1) and the Wave 6 dependent variable (i.e., DRUG at Wave 6).

* $p < .05$; ** $p < .01$.

Cross-sectional psychosocial correlates of substance use

Before reporting the relationships between different predictors and substance use, descriptive statistics of each of the variables under study are summarized in Table 11. For continuous variables, means and standard deviations are reported; for categorical variables, numbers and percentages of participants in each category are presented. Pearson's correlation coefficients among all continuous variables at each wave are also calculated and presented in Table 12.

Cross-sectional relationships between participants' use of substance and different predictors were examined at both Wave 1 and Wave 6. Tables 13 and14 show the results of logistic regression coefficients, Wald test, p value, and odds ratio for each of the predictors. It can be seen that results obtained from the two waves of data are quite consistent.

For Wave 1 data, age ($B = 0.23$, $p = 0.00$), gender ($B = 0.17$, $p = 0.01$), parental marital status (P1: $B = 0.28$, $p = 0.01$; P2: $B = 0.39$, $p = 0.01$; P3: $B = 0.34$, $p = 0.02$; P4: $B = 0.49$, $p = 0.00$), family life satisfaction ($B = -0.12$, $p = 0.00$), academic school competence ($B = -0.29$, $p = 0.00$), positive attributes ($B = -0.18$, $p = 0.00$), and general positive youth development qualities ($B = -0.36$, $p = $

Table 13. Predicting Drug use from personal and family factors, and positive youth development (Wave 1 Cross-Sectional)

	Predictor	B	Wald X^2	p	Odds Ratio (OR)	95% C.I. for OR Lower	95% C.I. for OR Upper
First Block	Age	0.23	54.85	0.00	1.25	1.18	1.33
	Gender	0.17	7.96	0.01	1.18	1.05	1.32
Second Block	FES	-0.04	0.24	0.62	0.96	0.82	1.13
	PMS: P1	0.28	6.68	0.01	1.32	1.07	1.63
	P2	0.39	7.24	0.01	1.48	1.11	1.97
	P3	0.34	5.27	0.02	1.40	1.05	1.86
	P4	0.49	12.59	0.00	1.63	1.24	2.12
	<u>FLS</u>	-0.12	13.69	0.00	<u>0.89</u>	0.83	0.94
Third Block	<u>ASC</u>	-0.29	33.41	0.00	<u>0.75</u>	0.68	0.83
	CBC	0.10	1.80	0.18	1.11	0.95	1.29
	<u>PA</u>	-0.18	11.12	0.00	<u>0.84</u>	0.75	0.93
	<u>GPYDQ</u>	-0.36	14.93	0.00	<u>0.70</u>	0.58	0.84
	PIT	0.09	2.69	0.10	1.09	0.98	1.20

Note: For dependent variable, 0 = never used any type of substance in the past half year; 1 = used substance at least once or twice in the past half year.
N = 6902. Goodness of fit test: Hosmer and Lemeshow Test X^2 = 9.51, df = 8, p = 0.30. Variables marked in bold are risk factors; variables underlined are protective factors.
FES = Family Economic Status; PMS = Parental Marital Status (P1 = Divorced but not remarried; P2 = Separate; P3 = Divorced and remarried; P4 = Other situations); FLS = Family Life Satisfaction; ASC = Academic and School Competence; CBC = Cognitive Behavioral Competence; PA = Prosocial Attributes; PIT = Positive Identity; GPYDQ = General Positive Youth Development Qualities.

0.00) were significant predictors, with the first three variables increasing the probability of using substance (risk factors) while the last four variables decreasing the likelihood of taking drugs (protective factors).

The odds ratios for the risk factors were 1.25 (age), 1.18 (gender), 1.32 (P1), 1.48 (P2), 1.40 (P3), and 1.63 (P4). This means that (1) while age increased one year, the participant would be 1.25 times more likely to take drugs; (2) male students were 1.18 times more likely to exhibit substance use behaviors than female students; and (3) the probability of taking drug in adolescents who had non-intact parental marital status was 1.32 to 1.63 times higher than that in

Table 14. Predicting Drug use from personal and family factors, and positive youth development (Wave 6 Cross-Sectional)

	Predictor	B	Wald X^2	p	Odds Ratio (OR)	95% C.I. for OR Lower	95% C.I. for OR Upper
First Block	Age	0.09	13.93	0.00	1.10	1.04	1.15
	Gender	0.11	4.12	0.04	1.11	1.00	1.24
Second Block	FES	-0.15	2.86	0.09	0.86	0.73	1.02
	PMS: P1	0.27	8.12	0.00	1.31	1.09	1.58
	P2	0.35	4.55	0.03	1.41	1.03	1.94
	P3	0.33	6.97	0.01	1.39	1.09	1.77
	P4	0.45	9.97	0.00	1.56	1.19	2.07
	FLS	-0.06	3.30	0.07	0.94	0.89	1.01
Third Block	ASC	-0.33	64.74	0.00	0.72	0.67	0.78
	CBC	0.12	2.45	0.12	1.12	0.97	1.30
	PA	-0.18	11.76	0.00	0.84	0.76	0.93
	GPYDQ	-0.15	2.71	0.10	0.87	0.73	1.03
	PIT	0.07	2.12	0.15	1.08	0.98	1.19

Note: For dependent variable, 0 = never used any type of substance in the past half year; 1 = used substance at least once or twice in the past half year.
N = 6330. Goodness of fit test: Hosmer and Lemeshow Test X^2= 12.39, df = 8, p =0.13. Variables marked in bold are risk factors; variables underlined are protective factors.
FES = Family Economic Status; PMS = Parental Marital Status (P1 = Divorced but not remarried; P2 = Separate; P3 = Divorced and remarried; P4 = Other situations); FLS = Family Life Satisfaction; ASC = Academic and School Competence; CBC = Cognitive Behavioral Competence; PA = Prosocial Attributes; PIT = Positive Identity; GPYDQ = General Positive Youth Development Qualities.

adolescents with intact families. For the protective factors, odds ratios were 0.89 for family life satisfaction, 0.75 for academic school competence, 0.84 for prosocial attributes, and 0.70 for general positive youth development qualities. These results suggest that participants who scored higher on the four positive youth development scales would be less likely to show substance use behaviors.

Similar results were obtained from the Wave 6 data. While old age, being male, and non-intact parental marital status predicted high probability of taking drug in the participants; higher scores on academic and school competence and prosocial attributes were related to decreased likelihood that the adolescent would display substance use behaviors.

Longitudinal correlates of substance abuse

To further examine whether individual characteristics, family factors, positive youth development constructs and perceived academic and school performance would contribute to adolescent substance use behaviors longitudinally, another logistic regression analysis was performed in which predictors measured at Wave 1 were used to predict the dependent variable (drug use behavior) measured at Wave 6. Participants' drug use behavior measured at Wave 1 was also entered in the model in order to control for the effects of one's initial drug use status on his/her later behaviors. Results of the logistic regression analysis are presented in Table 15. As shown in the table, adolescents who displayed substance use behaviors at Wave 1 were 4.63 times more likely to take drug at Wave 6 than those without such behavior at the initial status. Second, after controlling for the effects of initial substance abuse, participants' scores on academic and school competence and general positive youth qualities at Wave 1 significantly predicted the likelihood of taking drug at Wave 6. The higher the scores on the two high-order positive youth development constructs, the less likely the participants would display substance use behaviors. This finding further confirmed the cross-sectional results reported earlier that academic school competence and general positive youth development qualities were protective factors that prevent adolescents from using drugs. Third, participants whose parents were divorced and not remarried at Wave 1 were 1.29 times more likely than participants with parents who were in their first marriage to show substance use at Wave 6. Unexpectedly, the odds ratio was 1.18 for positive identity, meaning that adolescents who scored higher on positive identity scale at Wave 1 were more likely to take drug at Wave 6. Given that positive identity is an important construct of positive youth development, this finding was not consistent with the initial expectation.

Table 15. Predicting drug use from personal and family factors, and positive youth development (Wave 1→ Wave 6 Longitudinal)

	Predictor	B	Wald X^2	p	Odds Ratio (OR)	95% C.I. for OR Lower	95% C.I. for OR Upper
First Block	**Drug (Wave 1)**	1.53	431.06	0.00	4.63	4.01	5.35
Second Block	Age	0.01	0.01	0.98	1.00	0.93	1.08
	Gender	0.05	0.64	0.42	1.05	0.93	1.19
Third Block	FES	-0.18	3.48	0.06	0.84	0.69	1.01
	PMS:P1	0.26	3.82	0.05	1.29	1.00	1.67
	P2	0.00	0.00	0.99	1.00	0.68	1.47
	P3	0.19	1.18	0.28	1.21	0.86	1.73
	P4	0.10	0.37	0.54	1.10	0.80	1.54
	FLS	-0.04	1.50	0.22	0.96	0.90	1.02
Fourth Block	<u>ASC</u>	-0.23	16.30	0.00	<u>0.80</u>	0.71	0.89
	CBC	0.04	0.18	0.67	1.04	0.87	1.24
	PA	0.11	2.91	0.09	1.11	0.98	1.26
	<u>GPYDQ</u>	-0.37	11.51	0.00	<u>0.69</u>	0.56	0.86
	PIT	0.17	8.08	0.00	1.18	1.05	1.33

Note: For dependent variable, 0 = never used any type of substance in the past half year; 1 = used substance at least once or twice in the past half year.
N = 4738. Goodness of fit test: Hosmer and Lemeshow Test X^2= 3.80, df = 8, p = 0.88 Variables marked in bold are risk factors; variables underlined are protective factors. FES = Family Economic Status; PMS = Parental Marital Status (P1 = Divorced but not remarried; P2 = Separate; P3 = Divorced and remarried; P4 = Other situations); FLS = Family Life Satisfaction; ASC = Academic and School Competence; CBC = Cognitive Behavioral Competence; PA = Prosocial Attributes; PIT = Positive Identity; GPYDQ = General Positive Youth Development Qualities; DRUG (Wave 1) = Composite score of substance use at Wave 1.

DISCUSSION

While the prevalence of substance use found in the present study is basically consistent with those in the school survey reports by CRDA (5), there are several distinguishing features of this study. First, a broad range of substances were investigated in the present study, including both legal substances (such as tobacco and alcohol) and illicit drugs (e.g., psychotropic drugs and heroin). Second, while most tobacco or alcohol users reported taking the substances occasionally (once to twice in the past half year), for those reported using psychotropic drugs or heroin, a large proportion of them appeared to be frequent users. This indicates that there might be important differences between adolescents who reported smoking or drinking and those who took illicit drugs. As such, it would be interesting to compare the characteristics of the two groups in future study. Third, the longitudinal design of the present study would make it possible to examine the developmental trajectory of different substance use behaviors over time, though the discussion of this issue is beyond the scope of this paper.

Consistent with our first hypothesis, the analyses based on cross-sectional data at both Wave 1 (odds ratio = 1.18) and Wave 6 (odds ratio = 1.11) suggested that male adolescents were more likely than female adolescents to take drugs. Several theories are often used to explain gender difference in drug use. For example, there are views suggesting that female adolescents have a higher perceived risk of substance abuse than male adolescents, and thus are less likely to use drug. More recently, Svensson (28) proposed that gender difference in adolescent substance abuse can be understood in terms of parental monitoring and peer deviance. While boys are more prone to the exposure of deviant peers than are girls, girls are often more highly monitored than boys. As male adolescents appear to be a more vulnerable group for drug use, more preventive strategies that target at this population are in need.

With regard to the relationships between different family factors and drug use behaviors, the hypothesis that non-intact family status may serve as a risk factor for youth substance use was supported by the present results. Analyses based on both cross-sectional and longitudinal data showed that adolescents who lived in non-intact family (i.e., marital status of parents was divorced, separate, remarried or other situations) were more likely to report drug use behaviors than adolescents with intact family (i.e., parents were in their first marriage). As noted, adolescents living in the non-intact families may experience parental absence, both psychologically and physically. Besides, lack of parental supervision and dysfunctional family process are more often observed in non-intact families than in intact families. All these factors may contribute to adolescent substance use.

On the other hand, family economic status failed to predict substance use, meaning that poor adolescents did not show more substance use behaviors than adolescents from rich families. There are three possible reasons. First, adolescents living in poverty may not be able to afford the money to buy cigarette, alcohol, or other illicit drugs. Second, although poverty may produce negative beliefs, attitudes, and conditions that linked to drug use, poverty itself may not be directly associated with drug use. Third, while poverty is a multidimensional conception (e.g., income, education attainment; employment, and neighborhood), only one item was used to measure family economic status in the present study. In fact, another factor, family life satisfaction, was also assessed by one item asking the participants to rate their perceived satisfaction about family life on a Likert scale. It was found that although family life satisfaction significantly predicted drug use behavior at Wave 1, this relationship was found to be non-significant at Wave 6 and also in the longitudinal model. Obviously, the use of single item in measuring complicated constructs may decrease the power of the analyses.

As with prior research, the current study also found that adolescents who scored higher on different positive youth development constructs (academic social competence, prosocial attributes, and general positive youth development qualities) were less likely to take drugs than those with lower scores. These findings not only suggest that positive youth development is a protective factor for adolescent drug use, but also provide evidence for the effectiveness of the Project P.A.T.H.S. Based on the same sample of students, previous studies have reported that participants who attended the Project P.A.T.H.S. displayed higher levels of positive youth development while less problem behaviors (including substance use), as compared to students without joining the project (23,24). However, the question of whether the reduction of risk behaviors in the project participants is due to the enhancement of different positive youth development constructs in these students is not thorough addressed. The significant relationship between positive youth development constructs and the likelihood of taking substances found in the present study provides a preliminary but positive answer to this question. To further examine the role of different positive youth development constructs in preventing adolescent substance use, more in-depth studies are needed, although there are some initial findings suggesting that life satisfaction mediates the effect of positive youth development on adolescent problem behavior.

Nevertheless, the positive association between positive identity and substance use behavior found in this study was unexpected. In the present study, "positive identity" was measured by twelve items that capture both the participant's self identity and their future expectations. Previous research has demonstrated that both "clear and positive identity" and "positive belief in the future" predict better social and emotional adjustment and act as a protective factor in reducing the negative effect of high stress on self-rated competence (13,29). However, the longitudinal results in this study showed that participants who scored higher on positive identity at Wave 1 were more likely to report substance use behaviors than those scored lower on this construct. There are several possible explanations for this finding. The first explanation may be related to the measurement of substance use. Although different types of substance use were measured in this study, only the composite score (by averaging item scores) was employed in the regression analyses. This made it impossible to differentiate legal substance users (e.g., drinking alcohol) and illicit drug users. While it is obvious that using illicit drugs in Hong Kong society are viewed negative, alcohol use is perceived as basically normal and often accompanying with happy events. Therefore, for adolescents, occasional drinking may be considered as simply an attempt for new things. Compared to students with less positive views about themselves, students with clear and positive identity usually have more confidence in trying new things, and thus they may also be more willing to try alcohol or tobacco. This possibility may be examined in future studies by testing the relationships between positive identity and different substance use behaviors.

A second factor that could explain the unexpected finding may be that those youth who had high positive identity were those reaching puberty before other students. There are research findings showing that early pubertal timing is associated with the initiation of substance use (30-32). For example, Weisner and Ittel found that early maturing students reported a higher frequency of substance use (especially cigarette smoking) than did other students within the following years (19). The third possible explanation is related to studies that show aggressive children have inflated self-perception relative to non-aggressive children, and this inflated self-perception serves as a risk factor for increased problem behavior (33). It is possible that delinquent youth are overly confident in themselves, and this overconfidence leads to increases in aggression, delinquency, and substance use. Future studies may employ other indirect measures of positive identity, such as implicit association test, to avoid the influence of such bias in self-reported data.

Consistent with the literature, the present findings showed that perceived academic and school competence was negatively related to adolescent substance use. Theoretically, this finding gives support to the positive youth development literature that good academic and school performance is an internal asset which protects young people from risk behavior. Practically, how to help students with poor academic and school performance to stay away from drugs is an important issue to be considered. This is a particular thorny question for Hong Kong people because morbid emphasis on academic excellence is a significant characteristic of Hong Kong parenting.

In summary, the present study examined the current status of substance use among Hong Kong adolescents based on a large longitudinal sample of secondary school students. Several correlates of youth substance use in terms of gender, family factors, and positive youth development were also identified. The current results may inform further study on preventing youth substance abuse in Hong Kong. As Shek (4) noted, it is important to understand how different ecological factors may lead to adolescent substance abuse behaviors. Based on this ecological view, a "holistic development" approach that considers both risk and protective factors must be adopted in developing prevention strategies and programs for adolescents. In addition, as part of the Project P.A.T.H.S., the present study provides further evidence for the effectiveness of the program and suggests that promoting positive youth development could be a direction for the prevention of adolescent substance use in the future. The present results echo those findings suggesting that positive youth development reduces adolescent problem behavior, possibly via the impact of life satisfaction (34).

ACKNOWLEDGMENTS

The preparation for this paper and the Project P.A.T.H.S. were financially supported by The Hong Kong Jockey Club Charities Trust.

REFERENCES

[1] Substance Abuse and Mental Health Services Administration. Results from the 2009 national survey on drug use and health: Volume I. Summary of national findings. Rockville, MD: Office of Applied Studies; 2010.
[2] Arteaga I, Chen CC, Reynolds AJ. Childhood predictors of adult substance abuse. Child Youth Serv. Rev. 2010; 32(8):1108-20.

[3] Adesola A. Time to act. Drug Salvation Force 1998; 2(3):49.
[4] Shek DTL. Tackling adolescent substance abuse in Hong Kong: where we should and should not go. Scientific World Journal 2007;7:2021-30.
[5] Narcotics Division. The 2008/09 survey of drug use among students.Hong Kong: Narcotics Division, 2010.
[6] Bronfenbrenner U. The ecology of humandevelopment: Experiments by nature and design. Cambridge, MA: Harvard Univ Press, 1979.
[7] Brewer DD, Hawkins JD, Catalano RF, Neckerman HJ. Preventing serious, violent, and chronic juvenile offending: areview of selected strategies in childhood, adolescence, and the community. In: Howell JC, Krisberg B, Hawkins JD, Wilson JJ, eds. A sourcebook: Serious, violent, and chronic juvenile offenders.Thousand Oaks, CA: Sage, 1995:61-141.
[8] Farrington DP. The explanation and prevention of youthful offending. In: Hawkins JD, ed. Delinquency and crime: Current theories. New York: Cambridge Univ Press, 1996:68-148.
[9] Elliott DS, Huizinga D, Menard S. Multiple problem youth: Delinquency, substance use and mental healthproblems. New York: Springer, 1989.
[10] Hindelang MJ, Hirschi T, Weis JG. Measuring delinquency. Beverly Hills, CA: Sage, 1981.
[11] Weissberg RP, Caplan M, Harwood RL. Promoting competent young people in competence enhancing environments: asystems-based perspective on primary prevention. J. Consult. Clin. Psychol. 1991;59:830-41.
[12] Felner RD, Felner TY. Primary prevention programs in the educational context: a transactional ecological framework and analysis. In: Bond LA, Compas BE, eds.Primary prevention and promotion in the schools. Newbury, CA: Sage, 1989:13-49.
[13] Catalano RF, Berglund ML, Ryan JAM, Lonczak HS, Hawkins JD. Positive youth development in the United States: research findings on evaluations of positive youth development programs. Prev. Treat. 2002;25:1-111.
[14] Scales PC, Leffert N. Developmental assets:A synthesis of the scientific research on adolescent development. Minneapolis, MN: Search Institute, 1999.
[15] Wilson SJ, Lipsey M. The effects of school-based social information processing interventions on aggressive behavior, part I: universal programs. Campbell Syst. Rev. 2006;5.
[16] Tremblay RE, Kurtz L, Masse LC, Vitaro F, Pihl RO. A bi-modal preventive intervention for disruptive kindergarten boys: its impact through mid-adolescence. J. Consult. Clin. Psychol. 1995;63:560-8.
[17] Hawkins JW, Brown EC, Oesterle S, Arthur MW, Abbott RD, Catalano RF. Early effects of Communities That Care on targeted risks and initiation of delinquent behavior and substance use. J. Adolesc. Health 2008;43:15-22.
[18] Shek DTL, Ma HK, Merrick J, eds. Positive youth development: Development of a pioneering program in a Chinese context. London: Freund, 2002.
[19] Shek DTL. Conceptual framework underlying the development of a positive youth development program in Hong Kong.Int. J. Adolesc. Med. Health 2006;18:303-14.
[20] Shek DTL. Effectiveness of the Tier 1 Program of Project P.A.T.H.S.: findings based on the first 2 years of program implementation. Scientific World Journal 2009;9:539-47.

[21] Shek DTL, Ma HK. Editorial: evaluation of the Project P.A.T.H.S. in Hong Kong: are the findings replicable across different populations? Scientific World Journal 2010;10:178-81.
[22] Shek DTL, Sun RCF. Effectiveness of the Tier 1 Program of Project P.A.T.H.S.: findings based on three years of program implementation. Scientific World Journal 2010;10:1509-19.
[23] Shek DTL, Yu L. Prevention of adolescent problem behavior: longitudinal impact of the Project P.A.T.H.S. in Hong Kong. Scientific World Journal2011;11:546-67.
[24] Shek DTL, Ma CMS. Impact of the Project P.A.T.H.S. in the junior secondary school years: individual growth curve analyses. Scientific World Journal2011;11:253-66.
[25] Shek DTL, Siu AMH, Lee TY, Cheung CK, Chung R. Effectiveness of the Tier 1 Program of the Project P.A.T.H.S.: objective outcome evaluation based on a randomized group trial. Scientific World Journal 2008;8:4-12.
[26] Shek DTL, Chan YK, Lee P. Special issue on quality of life research in Chinese, Western and global contexts. Soc. Indic. Res. 2005;71:1-539.
[27] Shek DTL, Ma CMS. Dimensionality of the Chinese Positive Youth Development Scale: confirmatory factor analyses. Soc. Indic. Res. 2010;98:41-59.
[28] Svensson R. Gender differences in adolescents drug use: the impact of parental monitoring and peer deviance. Youth Soc. 2003;34:300-29.
[29] Wyman PA, Cowen EL, Work WC, Kerley JH. The role of children's future expectations in self-esteem functioning and adjustment to life stress: aprospective study of urban at-risk children. Special Issue: Milestones in the development of resilience. Dev. Psychopathol. 1993;5:649-61.
[30] Wiesner M, Ittel A. Relations of pubertal timing and depressive symptoms to substance use in early adolescence. J. Early Adolescence 2002;22:5-23.
[31] Dick DM, Rose RJ, Viken RJ, Kaprio J. Pubertal timing and substance use: associations between and within families across late adolescence. Dev. Psychol. 2000;36:180-9.
[32] Tschann JM, Adler NE, Irwin CE, Millstein SG, Turner RA, Kegeles SM. Initiation of substance use in early adolescence: the roles of pubertal timing and emotional distress. Health Psychol. 1994;13:326-33.
[33] Hughes JN, Cavell TA, Grossman PB. A positive view of self: riskor protection for aggressive children? Dev. Psychopathol. 1997;9:75-94.
[34] Sun RCF, Shek DTL. Life satisfaction, positive youth development, and problem behaviour among Chinese adolescents in Hong Kong. Soc. Indic. Res. 2010;95:455-74.

SECTION TWO: WHERE SHOULD WE GO FROM HERE?

In: Drug Abuse in Hong Kong
Editors: D Shek, R Sun and J Merrick
ISBN: 978-1-61324-491-3
©2012 Nova Science Publishers, Inc.

Chapter 12

TACKLING ADOLESCENT SUBSTANCE ABUSE IN HONG KONG: WHERE WE SHOULD GO AND SHOULD NOT GO?

Daniel TL Shek[1,a,b,c,d,e]

[a]Department of Applied Social Sciences,
The Hong Kong Polytechnic University, Hong Kong, PRC
[b]Public Policy Research Institute,
The Hong Kong Polytechnic University, Hong Kong, PRC
[c]East China Normal University, Shanghai, PRC
[d]Kiang Wu Nursing College of Macau, Macau, PRC
[e]Division of Adolescent Medicine, Department of Pediatrics,
Kentucky Children's Hospital, University of Kentucky,
College of Medicine, Lexington, Kentucky, US

ABSTRACT

In the 2007 Policy Address, the Chief Executive of the Hong Kong Special Administrative Region, PRC expressed the Administration's concern about adolescent substance abuse and proposed to form a high-level inter-departmental task force to tackle the problem in a holistic manner. In this

---

[1]Correspondence: Professor Daniel TL Shek, PhD, FHKPS, BBS, JP, Chair Professor, Department of Applied Social Sciences, The Hong Kong Polytechnic University, Hunghom, Hong Kong. E-mail: daniel.shek@polyu.edu.hk.

paper, the author presents his observations about adolescent substance abuse in Hong Kong and outlines the risk factors and related strategies based on the ecological perspective that the Government should consider in tackling the problem of adolescent substance abuse in Hong Kong. Furthermore, the directions that the Government should go and should not go are discussed.

INTRODUCTION

A survey of the websites of several international organizations (e.g., Office on Drugs and Crime of the United Nations, International Narcotics Control Board, National Institute of Drug Abuse in the United States, and European Monitoring Center for Drugs and Drug Addiction) shows that illicit drug use is a thorny global problem to be resolved. Probably because of the influence of popular culture and youth sub-culture, substance abuse among young people has also become an acute global problem. As Hong Kong is an international city where information flow (including those related to psychotropic drugs) is very quick, adolescent substance abuse is also a grave concern for Hong Kong (1, 2).

An examination of the substance abuse figures in the past twenty years showed that there were two peaks in the figures reported to the Central Registry of Drug Abuse (CRDA) maintained by the Narcotics Division of the Government. The first peak was in mid-1990s which was mainly related to easy access to tranquilizers which were not tightly controlled by legislations. The second peak was in early 2000s which was closely related to the rave party culture. In fact, these peaks mirrored the global trend of abusing non-opiate psychotropic substances and the growing belief among young people that psychotropic substance abuse is non-addictive and it is a valid choice of life (3).

Judging from the figures reported to the CRDA in recent years (seeTable 1), it is clear that the present moment is not the worst time for Hong Kong in terms of adolescent substance abuse. In fact, this situation can be attributed to the multi-prolonged approach adopted by the Narcotics Division and the Action Committee against Narcotics of the Government of the Hong Kong Special Administrative Region, PRC in the past years. Nevertheless, although figures on adolescent substance abusers reported to the Central Registry of Drug Abuse presented in Table 1 appeared to stabilize and decline in recent years, there are several observations that deserve our attention. First, as shown in Table 2, drugs abused by young people under the age of 21 were mainly psychotropic substances, particularly ketamine. Actually, ketamine abuse in Hong Kong could be regarded as quite unique because this drug is not commonly abused in other parts of the world. Second, with the return of Hong Kong to China in 1997, traveling between Hong Kong and Shenzhen in mainland China has become very popular, hence creating the problem of cross-border adolescent substance abuse. Actually, with the use of electronic home-return permits, adolescents can easily go back to Shenzhen to abuse drugs without leaving any trace in their travel documents. Hence, it is extremely difficult for parents to know whether their children have returned to Shenzhen. Finally, as the Hong Kong police force has stepped up action against adolescent substance abuse in rave parties, the venues of drug abuse among young people has become more diversified. Actually, some research studies showed that adolescents abused drugs in their homes, an emerging trend that deserves our attention (4).

Against this background, in his 2007 Policy Address, the Chief Executive of the Government of the Hong Kong Special Administrative Region voiced his concern about adolescent substance abuse in Hong Kong in Paragraph 86 of the Address, which states that "Hong Kong and many other advanced cities face similar social problems, among which youth drug abuse figures prominently. A lack of awareness, coupled with peer influence and curiosity, has led many young people to believe that taking psychotropic drugs is not that serious or even trendy. Drug abuse is dangerous to health as well as a criminal offence. I am deeply concerned about the problem of juvenile drug abuse because young people are the pillars of our future. We must tackle this issue with a multi-pronged approach. Otherwise, our society will definitely pay a high price in the future. To this end, I will appoint the Secretary for Justice, the incumbent Deputy Chairman of the Fight Crime Committee, to lead a high level inter-departmental task force which will make use of the existing anti-crime and anti-narcotics networks to consolidate strategies to combat juvenile drug abuse from a holistic perspective. The task force's terms of reference covers a wide range of areas, such as preventive education and publicity, treatment and rehabilitation, law enforcement, research and external co-operation. Task force members will do their best to mobilize various government departments and the local community to tackle juvenile drug abuse" (5).

How should the Hong Kong Government and community, particularly youth workers and researchers on adolescent substance abuse, respond to the Government's concern regarding tackling juvenile drug abuse? In this paper, three aspects of the issue are examined. First, ecological factors within the Hong Kong context that contribute to adolescent substance abuse are reviewed. Second, strategies and action plans based on the risk factors identified are examined.

Table 1. Substance abuse figures reported in the Central Registry of Drug Abuse

Year	1997	1998	1999	2000	2001	2002	2003	2004	2005	2006
All drug abusers	17,635	16,992	16,314	18,335	18,513	17,966	15,790	14,854	14,113	13,204
Mean age	34	34	35	32	33	34	34	35	35	34
Male	15,398	14,838	14,147	15,355	15,640	14,780	13,272	12,200	11,448	10,670
% of all	87.3	87.3	86.7	83.7	84.5	82.3	84.1	82.1	81.1	80.8
Mean age	35	35	36	34	34	35	36	36	37	36
Female	2,237	2,154	2,167	2,980	2,873	3,186	2,518	2,654	2,665	2,534
% of all	12.7	12.7	13.3	16.3	15.5	17.7	15.9	17.9	18.9	19.2
Mean age	27	27	28	25	26	27	28	28	28	27
Young persons aged under 21	3,150	2,841	2,482	4,020	3,902	3,002	2,207	2,186	2,276	2,549
% of all	17.9	16.7	15.2	21.9	21.1	16.7	14.0	14.7	16.1	19.3
Mean age	18	18	18	17	17	17	17	17	17	17
Newly reported persons	3,614	3,417	3,135	5,395	5,644	5,241	4,444	3,760	3,723	3,482
% of all	20.5	20.1	19.2	29.4	30.5	29.2	28.1	25.3	26.4	26.4
Mean age	24	24	25	23	23	24	25	24	23	23

Table 2. Type of drug abused in the Central Registry of Drug Abuse

	1997	1998	1999	2000	2001	2002	2003	2004	2005	2006
(1) Drug abusers with type of drugs reported										
No.	16,496	15,746	15,203	16,424	16,333	15,939	13,960	14,527	13,931	13,130
(2) Heroin abusers										
No.	14,291	13,588	13,003	12,188	11,575	11,826	10,357	10,147	9,757	8,101
% of (1)	86.6	86.3	85.5	74.2	70.9	74.2	74.2	69.8	70.0	61.7
(3) Psychotropic substance abusers										
No.	3,488	3,412	3,549	5,561	6,022	5,581	5,219	6,196	6,335	7,364
% of (1)	21.1	21.7	23.3	33.9	36.9	35.0	37.4	42.7	45.5	56.1
Ketamine abusers										
% of (1)	-	-	0.2	9.8	16.8	16.9	14.0	17.8	15.1	23.2
Triazolam/Midazolam/Zopiclone abusers										
% of (1)	5.9	5.7	6.1	5.6	5.5	7.8	11.2	12.1	14.6	16.9
Cannabis abusers										
% of (1)	8.0	8.9	8.5	8.7	7.5	8.1	7.5	7.7	8.2	7.4
MDMA (Ecstasy) abusers										
% of (1)	0.4	0.4	2.3	14.2	13.9	8.6	7.0	8.8	12.2	11.6
Methylamphetamine (Ice) abusers										
% of (1)	5.1	6.0	6.7	5.9	5.8	3.8	4.1	4.4	5.4	6.5
Cough medicine abusers										
% of (1)	2.7	1.8	1.9	1.9	1.8	2.4	3.9	4.5	5.1	5.7

Finally, the directions that the Government of Hong Kong Special Administrative Region should go and should not go regarding tackling adolescent substance abuse problems are discussed.

THE QUEST FOR AN ECOLOGICAL UNDERSTANDING OF ADOLESCENT SUBSTANCE ABUSE

At the very beginning, a proper understanding of the issue of adolescent substance abuse is in order. Although adolescent substance abuse can be understood in terms of different perspectives, the ecological perspective focusing on risk and protective factors has commonly been used to guide intervention strategies (6). There are numerous research studies showing that risk factors at the individual level (e.g., high sensation seeking, meaninglessness), family level (e.g., growing up in non-intact families), school level (e.g., low academic achievement, poor peer relationships) and community level (e.g., growing up in deprived communities) increase the chance of drug abuse in adolescents (7,8). On the other hand, there is also a vast literature showing that adolescents experiencing adversity do not necessarily end up in failures. Research findings showed that adolescents may adjust well despite the presence of adversity (9). According to Hauser (10), protective factors are "key constructs in conceptualizations of resilience" which "moderate the effects of individual vulnerabilities or environmental hazards, so that a given developmental trajectory reflects more adaptation in a given domain than would be the case if protective processes were not operating" (p.4). Based on a review of the resilience literature, Hauser (10) outlined several categories of protective factors, including individual (e.g., healthy attribution style, self-efficacy, hope, faith), relational (e.g., supportive home environment), community (e.g., good schools and other community assets) and general (e.g., good fortune) protective factors. In a review of stress, coping and resilience in children and youth, Smith and Carlson (11) similarly suggested that individual factors (e.g., optimism and faith), family factors(e.g., parental support and guidance), and external support systems (e.g., supportive non-parent adults) are important protective factors in children and adolescents experiencing environmental hazards. Utilizing research findings related to risk and protective processes in adolescent resilience, developers of positive youth development programs have attempted to reduce the impact of risk factors but promote the influence of protective factors via the developed programs. Historically, the utilization of risk and protective factors has shaped the "prevention science" perspective (12). Obviously, Hong Kong can learn much from this literature and devise relevant policies and services to tackle the problem of adolescent substance abuse, which is consistent with the "holistic perspective" emphasis in the 2007 Policy Address.

With reference to the research findings based on the ecological perspective, there are factors at different levels that contribute to the worrying adolescent substance abuse trend in Hong Kong. On the personal level, research findings showed that several factors predispose adolescent substance abuse problem. First, research findings have consistently showed that curiosity was a major factor leading to substance abuse among young people. Second, with material affluence and the rise of the number of nuclear families in Hong Kong, young people generally grow up without much turmoil. As such, they can be considered as growing up in "green house" where their relatively smooth upbringing would make them difficult to handle life adversities. Unfortunately, except some isolated effort, there are no systematic life skills and positive youth development programs in the formal curriculum in Hong Kong which help adolescents to cope with life adversities (13). Third, there are studies showing that a lack of life meaning is closely related to adolescent substance abuse. As Hong Kong has high social stress and there is a morbid emphasis on achievement (14), developing positive values in searching for life meaning may be difficult. Finally, adolescents with under-achievement and non-engagement (i.e., adolescents without study and work) are also prone to substance abuse (15).

There are two factors on the interpersonal system that increase the risk of adolescent substance abuse. First, the CRDA data have consistently showed that peer influence is a strong factor contributing to adolescent substance abuse. In fact, with the rapid growth of the youth sub-culture and intensification of virtual communication among young people (e.g., creating blogs that are only accessible by peers but not parents), undesirable peer influence is an important factor that may contribute to adolescent substance abuse (16). Second, with the growing number of nuclear families (i.e., families with few children) in Hong Kong, young people have fewer opportunities to practice interpersonal skills. Hence, they are easily susceptible to the influence of negative interpersonal experiences (e.g., conflict resolution and break up in love affairs) and they take drugs to cope with negative experiences associated with interpersonal difficulties.

There are several factors on the family level that are relevant to adolescent substance abuse in Hong Kong. First, with more parents working across the border, parenting in such families is weakened. Second, with reference to the rising number of cross-border marriages (old husband and young wife syndrome), adolescent children in such families are easily influenced by parental marital problems and parenting problems. Third, with the rise of divorce rates in the past

Table 3. Summary of ecological factors contributing to adolescent substance abuse in Hong Kong

Ecological System	Risk Factors
Personal	Curiosity
	Lack of psychosocial competencies and coping skills (growing up in "green house")
	Under-achievement
	Non-engagement
	Hopelessness, emptiness, and lack of life meaning
Interpersonal	Undesirable peer influence in relation to growing emphasis of peer recognition (e.g., blogs)
	Few siblings in the family to practice psychosocial skills (e.g., conflict resolution)
School	Under-achievement
	Undesirable after-school activities
Family	Cross-border working parents
	Cross-border marriages (old husband and young wife syndrome)
	Marital disruption and parental absence (both physically and psychologically)
	Loose parental supervision (morbid focus on academic excellence at the expense of value development)
	Acute decline in family solidarity
Societal	Growing addiction culture
	Postmodern youth culture
	Availability of drugs (light punishment for cases involving psychotropic substances); fine calculated in the cost of operating drug retailing business.
	Availability of drugs (cross-border consumption)
	Pathological emphasis on achievement leading to youth demoralization and mental health problems
	Growing poor adolescent population
	Growing pessimistic values and beliefs about having upward social mobility

decades, parental absence (both physically and psychologically) is a prominent problem in non-intact families. There are research findings showing that adolescent developmental outcomes are worse in non-intact families than in intact families. Fourth, there are research findings showing that parental supervision in adolescent children was loose (17, 18) and parents focus more on academic excellence at the expense of value development in adolescents (19). Finally, according to the social Development Index project undertaken by the Hong Kong Council of Social Service, there has been a substantial drop in family solidarity. As such, the problem of adolescent substance abuse should be understood in terms of a family perspective.

On the societal level, there are several indigenous factors that contribute to adolescent substance abuse in Hong Kong. First, besides substance abuse, the problems of pathological gambling (20) and net addiction (21) have become growing problems in Hong Kong. With the growing addiction culture which tends to create the false impression that addiction is basically not bad and normal, young people's attitudes to psychotropic drugs are adversely affected. Second, with the popularity of postmodern thoughts which posit that there is no absolute standard that differentiates "right" from "wrong", young people may simply think that substance abuse is a trendy lifestyle. Third, availability of drugs is a factor contributing to adolescent substance abuse. In particular, the light punishment for cases involving psychotropic drugs would not have deterring effects for the sellers. For example, some retailers of cough medicine abuse actually include the possible fine that they have to pay in their operating cost (4). Fourth, with convenient travel across the border, it is easy for young people to purchase and abuse drugs in the mainland with very low cost involved. In addition, the use of electronic home-return permits would make it virtually impossible for the parents to discover whether their children return to Shenzhen or not. Fifth, the growing poor population creates more poor adolescents who usually have limited opportunities for personal development and they are prone to academic under-achievement. Finally, growing pessimistic values and beliefs about having upward social mobility among the poor is a factor contributing to adolescent substance abuse. A summary of the risk factors that may contribute to adolescent substance abuse can be seen in Table 3.

STRATEGIES AND ACTION PLAN TO TACKLE THE PROBLEM

With reference to the factors that contribute to adolescent substance abuse problem, possible strategies that can be adopted to tackle adolescent substance abuse problem are summarized in Tables 4 and 5. There are several points in these two tables that deserve our attention. First, as there is no systematic positive youth development or drug prevention programs utilizing a curricular approach in the formal curriculum, and thus there is a great need to consider this issue. It should be noted that without systematic coverage of related topics in the curriculum, there is no guarantee that children and adolescents get adequate inoculation against substance abuse (6). Although the Narcotics Division conduct regular school talks, such talks are usually one-shot in nature and many schools simply express that their students do not have the need for substance abuse prevention. There are many studies in the West showing that effective substance abuse prevention programs can reduce substance abuse behavior in the program participants (22). As stated by Weissberg (23), successful positive youth development programs can improve the lives of millions of school children. As Hong Kong is an international city, the Hong Kong Government has to seriously consider implementing substance abuse prevention programs and/or positive youth development programs in a systematic and mandatory manner for children and adolescents in Hong Kong.

Second, it is obvious that there are many family factors contributing to substance abuse problems in young people. In fact, a review of both Western and Chinese literature shows that family factors, including systemic and dyadic parent-child factors, are related to adolescent delinquency and substance abuse (24). Moreover, healthy family conditions are social capital that can promote healthy adolescent development and protective factors that can help adolescents face adversity. Furthermore, morbid emphasis on academic achievement and relative negligence of the holistic development of children in contemporary Hong Kong culture (19) also deserves our attention of how such cultural attributes can be changed. Third, ecological analyses in Table 3 showed that factors at different levels are associated with adolescent drug abuse. The prevention implications of this analysis are that relevant factors on different levels should be included and it is rather futile to tackle adolescent substance abuse problem by simply changing factors at one level (e.g., increasing young people's knowledge about drugs and changing their attitudes at the personal level). Finally, prevention work at different levels, particularly secondary prevention and primary prevention, should be stepped up.

Obviously, different time frames and priorities would be involved in formulating policies and services based on the strategies outlined in Tables 4 and 5. Based on the above discussion, it is suggested that the following action plan should be considered:

- There is an urgent need to re-examine the sentencing guidelines for offences related to psychotropic substances to reflect the seriousness of the related offences.

- There is an urgent need to re-examine the immigration policy for allowing children under 18 to use the home-return permits to return to

Table 4. **Strategies with reference to the personal, interpersonal and family systems**

Ecological System	Risk Factors	Possible Strategy
Personal	Curiosity	Systematic drug education
	Lack of psychosocial competencies and coping skills (growing up in "green house")	Systematic and holistic positive youth development programs (which is severely lacking in the junior secondary school years)
	Under-achievement	Services focusing on creating success experiences for high-risk youth
	Non-engagement	Engagement services
	Hopelessness, emptiness, and lack of life meaning	Systematic and holistic positive youth development programs
Interpersonal	Undesirable peer influence in relation to growing emphases of peer recognition (e.g., blogs)	Systematic and holistic positive youth development programs
	Few siblings in family to practice psychosocial skills	Systematic and holistic positive youth development programs
School	Under-achievement	Creating success experiences for under-achievers
	Undesirable after-school activities	Meaningful after-school activities
Family	Cross-border working parents	Parenting education
	Cross-border marriages (old husband and young wife syndrome)	Fine-tuning of population policy; family life education
	Parental absence (both physically and psychologically)	Mentorship or surrogate parents; institutional care
	Loose parental supervision (morbid focus on academic excellence at the expense of value development)	Systematic parenting education
	Parental marital disruption	Mandatory parenting education for divorced cases
	Dropping of family solidarity	Strengthening family competence

Table 5. Strategies with reference to the social system

Ecological System	Risk Factors	Possible Strategy
Societal	Growing addiction culture (pathological gambling, net addiction, substance abuse)	Systematic drug education; positive youth development programs
	Growing poor population	Mandatory parenting education for CSSA recipients
	Growing pessimistic values and beliefs about having upward social mobility	Specialized positive youth development program; mentorship program; sub-cultural changes.
	Postmodern culture (e.g., youtube.com)	Anti-postmodern culture (e.g., godtube.com)
	Availability of drugs (light punishment for cases involving psychotropic substances); fine calculated in the cost of operating drug retailing business.	Revision of sentencing guidelines; stepping up law enforcement action.
	Availability of drugs (cross-border consumption)	Revision of immigration policy: parental consent must be sought for children under 18 to use home-return permits to return to China alone, particularly for cases under court orders and/or with previous addiction history.
	Pathological emphasis on achievement leading to youth demoralization and mental health problems	Community education; a new "cultural revolution" toward holistic development of young people; systematic positive youth development programs.

- China alone, particularly for cases under probation orders/care or protection orders and/or with previous drug addiction history.
- Systematic mechanisms related to early identification of adolescents with high risk for substance abuse should be devised in the family, school and community contexts.
- Proactive mechanisms for early identification of at-risk families (parental absence, families easily used by adolescents as venues for substance abuse) should be examined. Promotion of family competence and/or provision of alternative healthy family environment are possible

intervention directions that should be explored. As there is a lack of coordinated family policies in Hong Kong, it is a priority area that the Government should focus on in the near future.
- Promotion of parenting education in the general population and specialized parenting education for parents with special needs (e.g., CSSA families and single-parent families) regarding substance abuse prevention.
- The Government should seriously consider including systematic and universal drug education and positive youth development programs in the junior secondary school years. Without such inoculation effort, a wide range of adolescent developmental problems would emerge.
- Increase the number of social workers for schools admitting students with low academic achievement and schools in areas with high risk for substance abuse. Increase in police liaison officers in schools would also be helpful. Increase in professional manpower does make a difference in those needy schools.
- It is noteworthy that research on psychotropic substances abuse is severely lacking in the international and local contexts. Research findings are vital as far as evidence-based services and policy-formulation are concerned. As such, systematic research should be carried out.

DIRECTIONS THAT HONG KONG SHOULD GO AND SHOULD NOT GO

In devising policies for tackling adolescent substance abuse, the Government should carefully note that existing research findings have implications for the directions that Hong Kong should go as well as should not go. As shown in Table 6, the following directions should be avoided: a) research findings have shown that scary tactics do not work; b) blaming adolescents for their weaknesses alone do not work; c) understanding the problem from a single perspective does not help; d) formulation of policies and services with good intention only is futile; e) supply reduction cannot totally solve the problem because demand still exists; f) formulation of policies based on adults only will miss the viewpoints of young people; g) policies devised by the Government alone erodes the sense of ownership in different stakeholders, particularly in adolescents; and h) resources used mainly on treatment cannot help to tackle the problem of adolescent substance abuse. In contrast, the following directions should be considered by

Table 6. Directions that Hong Kong should go (and should not go) as far as strategies for tackling adolescent substance abuse is concerned

Direction that Hong Kong Should Not Go	Direction that Hong Kong Should Go
Scare adolescents	Understand adolescents
Blaming adolescents for their weaknesses	Understanding ecological factors leading to the problem
Understand the problem from a single perspective (e.g., personal problems)	Ecological understanding, particularly family-based intervention, is important
Formulation of services and policies with good will only	Evidence-based and research driven services and policies
Supply reduction strategies only	Supply reduction and demand reduction strategies
Services and policies involving adults only	Services and policies with the involvement of adults and adolescents
Policies devised by the Government alone	Policy-making involving stakeholders in different sectors
Resources mainly devoted to treatment	Resources devoted to primary, secondary and tertiary prevention

Hong Kong: a) while pointing out that adolescent substance abuse is a "problem", understanding adolescents is equally important; b) it is important to understand how different ecological factors lead to adolescent substance abuse; c) ecological understanding, particularly family-based intervention, is of paramount important; d) evidence-based and research driven services and policies should be desired for; e) supply reduction and demand reduction are equally important; f) involvement of adolescents in the process of formulating services and policies is important; g) policy-making involving stakeholders in different sectors is needed; and h) resources devoted to primary, secondary and tertiary prevention are equally important.

CONCLUSION

In conclusion, this paper argues for an ecological understanding of the phenomenon of adolescent substance abuse in Hong Kong so that a more holistic approach can be achieved. This approach is consistent with the spirit of "holistic perspective" as stated in the 2007 Policy Address of the Chief Executive of the Government of Special Administrative Region. I earnestly hope that through this paper, further discussion incorporating the concepts of risk factors, protective factors, at-risk families, ecological perspective, primary prevention, secondary prevention, tertiary prevention, positive youth development and holistic adolescent development in exploring a more long-term and coordinated approach in tackling adolescent substance abuse in Hong Kong will be carried out.

ACKNOWLEDGMENTS

The preparation for this paper was financially supported by the Wofoo Foundation Limited.

REFERENCES

[1] Shek DTL. International conference on tackling drug abuse: conference proceedings. Hong Kong: Narcotics Division, Security Bureau, Government of Hong Kong Special Administrative Region, 2006.
[2] Shek DTL. Adolescent developmental issues in Hong Kong: relevance to positive youth development programs in Hong Kong. Int. J. Adolesc. Med. Health 2006;18:341-54.
[3] Shek DTL. Tackling drug abuse in a changing world: challenges and responses. In: Shek DTL. International conference on tackling drug abuse: conference proceedings. Hong Kong: Narcotics Division, Security Bureau, 2006:3-9.
[4] Shek DTL, Lam CM. Adolescent cough medicine abuse in Hong Kong: implications for the design of positive youth development programs in Hong Kong. Int. J. Adolesc.Med. Health 2006;18:493-503.
[5] Legislative Council. Legislative Council meeting: official record of proceedings 2007 October 10. Government of Hong Kong Special Administrative Region of the People's Republic of China. Accessed 2011 Feb 11. Available at:http://www.legco.gov.hk/yr07-08/english/counmtg/hansard/cm1010-translate-e.pdf.
[6] Shek DTL. Conceptual framework underlying the development of a positive youth development program in Hong Kong. Int. J. Adolesc. Med. Health 2006;18:303-14.
[7] Weissberg RP, Caplan M, Harwood RL. Promoting competent young people in competence-enhancing environments: a systems-based perspective on primary prevention. J. Consult. Clin. Psychol. 1991;59:830-41.
[8] Felner RD, Felner TY. Primary prevention programs in the educational context: a transactional-ecological framework and analysis. In: Bond LA, Compas BE, eds. Primary prevention and promotion in the schools. Newbury, CA: Sage,1989:13-49.
[9] Shek DTL. Resilience in adolescence: western models and local findings. In: Chinese Y.M.C.A. of Hong Kong, ed. Centennial conference on counseling in China, Taiwan and Hong Kong. Hong Kong: Chinese Y.M.C.A. of Hong Kong, 2001:3-21.
[10] Hauser ST. Understanding resilient outcomes: adolescent lives across time and generations. J. Res. Adolesc. 1999;9:1-24.
[11] Smith C, Carlson BE. Stress, coping and resilience in children and youth. Soc. Serv. Rev. 1997;71(2):231-56.

[12] Tobler NS, Roona MR, Ochshorn P, Marshall DG, Streke AV, Stackpole KM. School-based adolescent drug prevention programs: 1998 meta-analysis. J. Prim. Prev. 2000;20:275-337.
[13] Shek DTL. Construction of a positive youth development program in Hong Kong. Int. J. Adolesc. Med. Health 2006;18:299-302.
[14] Shek DTL. Social stress in Hong Kong. In: Estes J, ed. Social development index. Hong Kong: Oxford University Press,2005:167-89.
[15] Shek DTL, Lee BM. "Non-engaged" young people in Hong Kong: key statistics and observations. Int. J. Adolesc. Med. Health 2004;16:145-63.
[16] Lam CM, Shek DTL. A qualitative study of cough medicine abuse among Chinese young people in Hong Kong. J. Subst. Abuse 2006;11:233-44.
[17] Shek DTL. Drop in family harmony in Hong Kong: an ecological analysis and related research. In: Shek DTL, ed. Conference on strengthening Hong Kong's families: awareness, commitment and action:conference proceedings. Hong Kong: Central Policy Unit, Government of Hong Kong Special Administrative Region, 2006 September 5.
[18] Shek DTL, Han XY, Lee BM. Perceived parenting patterns and parent-child relational qualities in adolescents in Hong Kong and Shanghai. Chin. J. Sociology 2006 26:137-57.
[19] Shek DTL, Chan LK. Hong Kong Chinese parents' perceptions of the ideal child. J. Psychol. 1999;133:291-302.
[20] Shek DTL, Yiu TLI, Chan MLE. Advances in problem gambling: theory, service and research in the Asia-Pacific region. Hong Kong: Tung Wah Group of Hospitals and Social Welfare Practice and Research Centre, Chinese University of Hong Kong, 2006.
[21] Tang MYV, Shek DTL, Working Group on Net Addiction. Net addiction and non-addiction: a report on youth characteristics. Hong Kong: Lutheran Ming Wah Integrated Youth Service, Hong Kong Lutheran Social Service, 2007.
[22] Catalano RF, Berglund ML, Ryan JAM, Lonczak HS, Hawkins JD. Positive youth development in the United States: research findings on evaluations of positive youth development programs. Ann. Am. Acad. of Polit. Soc. Sci. 2004;591:98-124.
[23] Weissberg RP. Improving the lives of millions of school children. Am. Psychol. 2000;55:1360-73.
[24] Shek DTL. Family processes and development outcomes in Chinese adolescents. Hong Kong J. Pediatrics 2004;9:316-24.

SECTION THREE: ACKNOWLEDGMENTS

In: Drug Abuse in Hong Kong
Editors: D Shek, R Sun and J Merrick

ISBN: 978-1-61324-491-3
©2012 Nova Science Publishers, Inc.

Chapter 13

ABOUT THE EDITORS

Daniel TL Shek[a,b,c,d,e], Rachel CF Sun[a] and Joav Merrick[e]
[a]Department of Applied Social Sciences,
The Hong Kong Polytechnic University, Hong Kong, PRC
[b]Public Policy Research Institute,
The Hong Kong Polytechnic University, Hong Kong, PRC
[c]East China Normal University, Shanghai, PRC
[d]Kiang Wu Nursing College of Macau, Macau, PRC
[e]Division of Adolescent Medicine, Department of Pediatrics,
Kentucky Children's Hospital, University of Kentucky,
College of Medicine, Lexington, Kentucky, US

Daniel TL Shek, PhD, FHKPS, BBS, JP, is Chair Professor of Applied Social Sciences, Department of Applied Social Sciences, Hong Kong Polytechnic University, Hunghom, Hong Kong, PRC;Advisory Professor of East China Normal University, Shanghai, PRC; Honorary Professor of Kiang Wu Nursing College of Macau, Macau, PRC; Adjunct Professor of Division of Adolescent Medicine, Department of Pediatrics, University of Kentucky, College of Medicine, USA. He is Chief Editor of *Journal of Youth Studies*, Consulting Editor of *Journal of Clinical Psychology*, international consultant of *American Journal of Family Therapy*, and editorial board member of *Social Indicators Research, International Journal of Adolescent Medicine and Health, The Scientific World Journal (Child Health and Human Development and Holistic Health and Medicine domains), Asian Journal of Counselling, International Journal of*

Disability and Human Development, and *Bentham Open Family Studies Journal.* He has served in many government advisory bodies, including the Action Committee against Narcotics, Commission on Youth, Fight Crime Committee and Family Council. He has published numerous books, book chapters and more than 300 scientific articles in international refereed journals. E-mail: daniel.shek@polyu.edu.hk

Rachel CF Sun, PhD, is Assistant Professor at the Faculty of Education, The University of Hong Kong, Hong Kong, PRC. She teaches in the areas of psychology of teaching and learning, and child and adolescent development. Her research areas include academic achievement motivation, student misbehavior, school satisfaction, life satisfaction, positive youth development, adolescent suicidal ideation, and psychological health. She is a co-principal investigator of a huge and pioneering positive youth development project in Hong Kong. She is an Executive Committee member of the Society of Boys' Centres, and a member of the Editorial Board of *Research on Social Work Practice.* E-mail: rachels@hku.hk.

Joav Merrick, MD, MMedSci, DMSc, is Professor of pediatrics, child health and human development affiliated with Kentucky Children's Hospital, University of Kentucky, Lexington, United States and the Pediatric Department, Mt Scopus Campus, Hadassah-Hebrew-University Medical Center, Jerusalem, Israel, the medical director of the Health Service, Division for Mental Retardation, Ministry of Social Affairs, Jerusalem, the founder and director of the National Institute of Child Health and Human Development. Numerous publications in the field of pediatrics, child health and human development, rehabilitation, intellectual disability, disability, health, welfare, abuse, advocacy, quality of life and prevention. Received the Peter Sabroe Child Award for outstanding work on behalf of Danish Children in 1985 and the International LEGO-Prize ("The Children's Nobel Prize") for an extraordinary contribution towards improvement in child welfare and well-being in 1987. E-mail: jmerrick@zahav.net.il

In: Drug Abuse in Hong Kong
Editors: D Shek, R Sun and J Merrick
ISBN: 978-1-61324-491-3
©2012 Nova Science Publishers, Inc.

Chapter 14

ABOUT THE DEPARTMENT OF APPLIED SOCIAL SCIENCES, THE HONG KONG POLYTECHNIC UNIVERSITY

Daniel TL Shek[a,b,c,d,e], Rachel CF Sun[a] and Joav Merrick[e]
[a]Department of Applied Social Sciences,
The Hong Kong Polytechnic University, Hong Kong, PRC
[b]Public Policy Research Institute,
The Hong Kong Polytechnic University, Hong Kong, PRC
[c]East China Normal University, Shanghai, PRC
[d]Kiang Wu Nursing College of Macau, Macau, PRC
[e]Division of Adolescent Medicine, Department of Pediatrics,
Kentucky Children's Hospital, University of Kentucky,
College of Medicine, Lexington, Kentucky, US

The Department of Applied Social Sciences (APSS) of The Hong Kong Polytechnic University is one of the largest and most vibrant centres in the region dedicated to the education and training of professional social workers, social policy and welfare administrators, psychologists and counselors in Hong Kong.

The Department started as the Institute of Social Work Training in 1973. It joined the Hong Kong Polytechnic in 1977 and became its School of Social Work. The School was eventually renamed the Department of Applied Social Sciences. APSS celebrated its 35th anniversary in the academic year of 2007/08.Currently there are 93 full-time academics, over 80 research/project staff, 20 fieldwork supervisors and 34 colleagues in other categories, including administrative and supporting personnel.

The Department has six thriving research centres: Centre for Social Policy Studies, China Research and Development Network, Network for Health and Welfare Studies, Professional Practice and Assessment Centre, Centre for Third Sector Studies, and the Manulife Centre for Children with Specific Learning Disabilities, providing platforms for collaborative research and practice projects with government departments and non-governmental organizations.

The Department of Applied Social Sciences offers taught programs in the fields of Social Work, Social Policy and Administration, Counseling, and Applied Psychology, as well as research degrees at MPhil and PhD levels. In 2008/09, APSS offered some 20 Programs for Higher Diploma, Degree, Postgraduate, MPhil and PhD students. There are currently about 1,500 students enrolled in the various APSS programs and we have graduated more than 14,000 students over the years.

In the past decade, the Department has successfully expanded into the Chinese mainland. The Department currently offers a MSW (China) Program in collaboration with Peking University and a Joint PolyU-PekingU Social Work Research Centre has been established to foster research in Social Work and Social Policy.

CONTACT

Professor Daniel TL Shek, PhD, FHKPS, BBS, JP
Chair Professor of Applied Social Sciences
Department of Applied Social Sciences
The Hong Kong Polytechnic University
Hunghom, Hong Kong
E-mail: daniel.shek@polyu.edu.hk

In: Drug Abuse in Hong Kong
Editors: D Shek, R Sun and J Merrick
ISBN: 978-1-61324-491-3
©2012 Nova Science Publishers, Inc.

Chapter 15

About the National Institute of Child Health and Human Development IN ISRAEL

Daniel TL Shek[a,b,c,d,e], Rachel CF Sun[a] and Joav Merrick[e]
[a]Department of Applied Social Sciences,
The Hong Kong Polytechnic University, Hong Kong, PRC
[b]Public Policy Research Institute,
The Hong Kong Polytechnic University, Hong Kong, PRC
[c]East China Normal University, Shanghai, PRC
[d]Kiang Wu Nursing College of Macau, Macau, PRC
[e]Division of Adolescent Medicine, Department of Pediatrics,
Kentucky Children's Hospital, University of Kentucky,
College of Medicine, Lexington, Kentucky, US

The National Institute of Child Health and Human Development (NICHD) in Israel was established in 1998 as a virtual institute under the auspices of the Medical Director, Ministry of Social Affairs and Social Services in order to function as the research arm for the Office of the Medical Director. In 1998 the National Council for Child Health and Pediatrics, Ministry of Health and in 1999 the Director General and Deputy Director General of the Ministry of Health endorsed the establishment of the NICHD.

MISSION

The mission of a National Institute for Child Health and Human Development in Israel is to provide an academic focal point for the scholarly interdisciplinary study of child life, health, public health, welfare, disability, rehabilitation, intellectual disability and related aspects of human development. This mission includes research, teaching, clinical work, information and public service activities in the field of child health and human development.

SERVICE AND ACADEMIC ACTIVITIES

Over the years many activities became focused in the south of Israel due to collaboration with various professionals at the Faculty of Health Sciences (FOHS) at the Ben Gurion University of the Negev (BGU). Since 2000 an affiliation with the Zusman Child Development Center at the Pediatric Division of Soroka University Medical Center has resulted in collaboration around the establishment of the Down Syndrome Clinic at that center. In 2002 a full course on "Disability" was established at the Recanati School for Allied Professions in the Community, FOHS, BGU and in 2005 collaboration was started with the Primary Care Unit of the faculty and disability became part of the master of public health course on "Children and society". In the academic year 2005-2006 a one semester course on "Aging with disability" was started as part of the master of science program in gerontology in our collaboration with the Center for Multidisciplinary Research in Aging.

RESEARCH ACTIVITIES

The affiliated staff have over the years published work from projects and research activities in this national and international collaboration. In the year 2000 the International Journal of Adolescent Medicine and Health and in 2005 the International Journal on Disability and Human development of Freund Publishing House (London and Tel Aviv), in the year 2003 the TSW-Child Health and Human Development and in 2006 the TSW-Holistic Health and Medicine of the Scientific World Journal (New York and Kirkkonummi, Finland), all peer-reviewed international journals were affiliated with the National Institute of Child

Health and Human Development. From 2008 also the International Journal of Child Health and Human Development (Nova Science, New York), the International Journal of Child and Adolescent Health (Nova Science) and the Journal of Pain Management (Nova Science) affiliated and from 2009 the International Public Health Journal (Nova Science) and Journal of Alternative Medicine Research (Nova Science).

NATIONAL COLLABORATIONS

Nationally the NICHD works in collaboration with the Faculty of Health Sciences, Ben Gurion University of the Negev; Department of Physical Therapy, Sackler School of Medicine, Tel Aviv University; Autism Center, Assaf HaRofeh Medical Center; National Rett and PKU Centers at Chaim Sheba Medical Center, Tel HaShomer; Department of Physiotherapy, Haifa University; Department of Education, Bar Ilan University, Ramat Gan, Faculty of Social Sciences and Health Sciences; College of Judea and Samaria in Ariel and recently also collaborations has been established with the Department of Pediatrics at Hadassah, Mt Scopus Campus, Center for Pediatric Chronic Illness, Hadassah-University Medical Center in Jerusalem.

INTERNATIONAL COLLABORATIONS

Internationally with the Department of Disability and Human Development, College of Applied Health Sciences, University of Illinois at Chicago; Strong Center for Developmental Disabilities, Golisano Children's Hospital at Strong, University of Rochester School of Medicine and Dentistry, New York; Centre on Intellectual Disabilities, University of Albany, New York; Centre for Chronic Disease Prevention and Control, Health Canada, Ottawa; Chandler Medical Center and Children's Hospital, Kentucky Children's Hospital, Section of Adolescent Medicine, University of Kentucky, Lexington; Chronic Disease Prevention and Control Research Center, Baylor College of Medicine, Houston, Texas; Division of Neuroscience, Department of Psychiatry, Columbia University, New York; Institute for the Study of Disadvantage and Disability, Atlanta; Center for Autism and Related Disorders, Department Psychiatry, Children's Hospital Boston, Boston; Department of Paediatrics, Child Health and

Adolescent Medicine, Children's Hospital at Westmead, Westmead, Australia; International Centre for the Study of Occupational and Mental Health, Düsseldorf, Germany; Centre for Advanced Studies in Nursing, Department of General Practice and Primary Care, University of Aberdeen, Aberdeen, United Kingdom; Quality of Life Research Center, Copenhagen, Denmark; Nordic School of Public Health, Gottenburg, Sweden, Scandinavian Institute of Quality of Working Life, Oslo, Norway; Centre for Quality of Life of the Hong Kong Institute of Asia-Pacific Studies and School of Social Work, Chinese University, Hong Kong.

TARGETS

Our focus is on research, international collaborations, clinical work, teaching and policy in health, disability and human development and to establish the NICHD as a permanent institute at one of the residential care centers for persons with intellectual disability in Israel in order to conduct model research and together with the four university schools of public health/medicine in Israel establish a national master and doctoral program in disability and human development at the institute to secure the next generation of professionals working in this often non-prestigious/low-status field of work. For this project we need your support. We are looking for all kinds of support and eventually an endowment.

CONTACT

Joav Merrick, MD, DMSc
Professor of Pediatrics, Child Health and Human Development
Medical Director, Division for Mental Retardation, Ministry of Social Affairs and Social Services, POB 1260, IL-91012 Jerusalem, Israel.
E-mail: jmerrick@inter.net.il

In: Drug Abuse in Hong Kong
Editors: D Shek, R Sun and J Merrick

ISBN: 978-1-61324-491-3
©2012 Nova Science Publishers, Inc.

Chapter 16

ABOUT THE BOOK SERIES "HEALTH AND HUMAN DEVELOPMENT"

Daniel TL Shek[a,b,c,d,e], Rachel CF Sun[a] and Joav Merrick[e]
[a]Department of Applied Social Sciences,
The Hong Kong Polytechnic University, Hong Kong, PRC
[b]Public Policy Research Institute,
The Hong Kong Polytechnic University, Hong Kong, PRC
[c]East China Normal University, Shanghai, PRC
[d]Kiang Wu Nursing College of Macau, Macau, PRC
[e]Division of Adolescent Medicine, Department of Pediatrics,
Kentucky Children's Hospital, University of Kentucky,
College of Medicine, Lexington, Kentucky, US

Health and human development is a book series with publications from a multidisciplinary group of researchers, practitioners and clinicians for an international professional forum interested in the broad spectrum of health and human development.

- Merrick J, Omar HA, eds. Adolescent behavior research. International perspectives. New York: Nova Science, 2007.
- Kratky KW. Complementary medicine systems: Comparison and integration. New York: Nova Science, 2008.
- Schofield P, Merrick J, eds. Pain in children and youth. New York: Nova Science, 2009.

- Greydanus DE, Patel DR, Pratt HD, Calles Jr JL, eds. Behavioral pediatrics, 3 ed. New York: Nova Science, 2009.
- Ventegodt S, Merrick J, eds. Meaningful work: Research in quality of working life.New York: Nova Science, 2009.
- Omar HA, Greydanus DE, Patel DR, Merrick J, eds. Obesity and adolescence. A public health concern. New York: Nova Science, 2009.
- Lieberman A, Merrick J, eds. Poverty and children. A public health concern. New York: Nova Science, 2009.
- Goodbread J. Living on the edge. The mythical, spiritual and philosophical roots of social marginality. New York: Nova Science, 2009.
- Bennett DL, Towns S, Elliot E, Merrick J, eds. Challenges in adolescent health: An Australian perspective. New York: Nova Science, 2009.
- Schofield P, Merrick J, eds. Children and pain. New York: Nova Science, 2009.
- Sher L, Kandel I, Merrick J. Alcohol-related cognitive disorders: Research and clinical perspectives. New York: Nova Science, 2009.
- Anyanwu EC. Advances in environmental health effects of toxigenic mold and mycotoxins. New York: Nova Science, 2009.
- Bell E, Merrick J, eds. Rural child health. International aspects. New York: Nova Science, 2009.
- Dubowitz H, Merrick J, eds. International aspects of child abuse and neglect.New York: Nova Science, 2010.
- Shahtahmasebi S, Berridge D. Conceptualizing behavior: A practical guide to data analysis.New York: Nova Science, 2010.
- Wernik U. Chance action and therapy. The playful way of changing. New York: Nova Science, 2010.
- Omar HA, Greydanus DE, Patel DR, Merrick J, eds. Adolescence and chronic illness. A public health concern. New York: Nova Science, 2010.
- Patel DR, Greydanus DE, Omar HA, Merrick J, eds. Adolescence and sports. New York: Nova Science, 2010.
- Shek DTL, Ma HK, Merrick J, eds. Positive youth development: Evaluation and future directions in a Chinese context. New York: Nova Science, 2010.
- Shek DTL, Ma HK, Merrick J, eds. Positive youth development: Implementation of a youth program in a Chinese context. New York: Nova Science, 2010.

About the book series "Health and Human Development" 227

- Omar HA, Greydanus DE, Tsitsika AK, Patel DR, Merrick J, eds. Pediatric and adolescent sexuality and gynecology: Principles for the primary care clinician.New York: Nova Science, 2010.
- Chow E, Merrick J, eds. Advanced cancer. Pain and quality of life. New York: Nova Science, 2010.
- Latzer Y, Merrick, J, Stein D, eds. Understanding eating disorders. Integrating culture, psychology and biology. New York: Nova Science, 2010.
- Sahgal A, Chow E, Merrick J, eds. Bone and brain metastases: Advances in research and treatment. New York: Nova Science, 2010.
- Postolache TT, Merrick J, eds. Environment, mood disorders and suicide. New York: Nova Science, 2010.
- Maharajh HD, Merrick J, eds. Social and cultural psychiatry experience from the Caribbean Region.New York: Nova Science, 2010.
- Mirsky J. Narratives and meanings of migration. New York: Nova Science, 2010.
- Harvey PW. Self-management and the health care consumer. New York: Nova Science, 2011.
- Ventegodt S, Merrick J. Sexology from a holistic point of view. New York: Nova Science, 2011.
- Ventegodt S, Merrick J. Principles of holistic psychiatry: A textbook on holistic medicine for mental disorders. New York: Nova Science, 2011.
- Greydanus DE, Calles Jr JL, Patel DR, Nazeer A, Merrick J, eds. Clinical aspects of psychopharmacology in childhood and adolescence. New York: Nova Science, 2011.
- Bell E, Seidel BM, Merrick J, eds. Climate change and rural child health.New York: Nova Science, 2011.
- Bell E, Zimitat C, Merrick J, eds. Rural medical education: Practical strategies. New York: Nova Science, 2011.
- Latzer Y, Tzischinsky. The dance of sleeping and eating among adolescents: Normal and pathological perspectives. New York: Nova Science, 2011.

CONTACT

Professor Joav Merrick, MD, MMedSci, DMSc
Medical Director, Health Services, Division for Mental Retardation

Ministry of Social Affairs, P.O. Box 1260
IL-91012 Jerusalem, Israel
E-mail: jmerrick@internet-zahav.net

SECTION FOUR: INDEX

INDEX

A

academic performance, 17, 31, 33, 203, 208
access, 4, 86, 234
accounting, 51
adaptation, 121, 240
adjustment, 6, 63, 81, 83, 194, 195, 225, 229
administrators, 32, 36, 41, 46, 261
adolescent development, 6, 14, 16, 17, 19, 28, 81, 88, 138, 161, 228, 243, 245, 249, 251, 258
adolescent drinking, 197
adolescent problem behavior, 181, 182, 196, 197, 224, 226, 228
adulthood, 82, 116, 135, 200
adults, xx, 17, 196, 241, 250
adverse effects, 7, 22
advocacy, 18, 258
affluence, 181, 241
age, 4, 5, 105, 128, 183, 192, 196, 203, 208, 209, 217, 218, 220, 235, 237, 238
agencies, 11, 14, 140
aggressive behavior, 228
alcohol use, 32, 192, 222, 225
alertness, 147
alienation, 167
American Civil Liberties Union, 29
anchoring, 163
ANCOVA analyses, 65, 67, 68, 69, 72, 73, 74, 75

arrests, 32
Asia, 8, 195, 203, 253, 266
assertiveness, 17
assessment, 43, 44, 45, 65, 99, 106, 116, 162, 175
assets, 19, 228, 240
Astro Teens programs, 89, 90, 106, 137, 140, 161
athletes, 28, 31, 34, 36, 37, 38, 39, 41, 42, 46, 52
atmosphere, 191
attribution, 240
audit, 51, 155
authority, 15, 24, 160
autonomy, 18
awareness, 23, 31, 35, 181, 200, 235, 253

B

base, 7, 8, 10, 12, 15, 17, 22, 23, 24, 25, 48, 50, 51, 80, 82, 83, 116, 117, 135, 140, 155, 160, 177, 228, 249, 251
base rate, 50
behavioral manifestations, 196
behaviors, 58, 63, 80, 151, 152, 153, 164, 191, 192, 193, 195, 200, 202, 203, 206, 208, 209, 210, 215, 218, 220, 222, 223, 224, 225, 226
beneficial effect, 152, 175

benefits, 7, 22, 31, 64, 69, 72, 78, 90, 99, 106, 123, 134, 140, 143, 155
bias, 47, 50, 89, 117, 156, 226
blogs, 242, 246
board members, 12, 61
bonding, 36, 61, 120, 182, 183, 187, 188, 189
brain, xx, xxi, 196, 271

C

cancer, 271
cannabis, 185, 189, 206, 212, 215
caregivers, 17
Caribbean, 271
case studies, 21, 139
categorization, 125, 126, 129, 130, 146, 147, 148
category a, 65, 217
causal interpretation, 49
challenges, 160, 161, 252
charitable organizations, 10
charities, xiii, 9, 11, 23, 117, 177
chemical, xix, xx, 120
Chicago, 265
child abuse, 270
child rearing, 14
childhood, 194, 227, 272
children, 5, 14, 61, 82, 88, 99, 105, 120, 161, 196, 225, 229, 235, 240, 242, 243, 244, 245, 246, 248, 252, 253, 270
China, xi, xx, 3, 4, 9, 27, 48, 57, 85, 103, 119, 137, 159, 179, 184, 194, 199, 233, 235, 248, 252, 257, 261, 262, 263, 269
Chinese Self-Esteem Scale, 65
chronic illness, 271
cigarette smoking, 225
CIPP model, 122, 135, 138, 140, 143, 157
cities, 235
classes, 21
classification, 93, 94, 98, 109, 113, 124, 125, 126, 129, 130, 132, 133, 146, 147, 148, 149, 152, 153
classroom, 19, 205
clients, 12, 89, 134, 164

coding, 92, 97, 110, 112, 113, 115, 123, 140, 142, 216
cognitive abilities, 17, 148
coherence, 153
collaboration, 141, 142, 262, 264, 265
common sense, 14
communication, 17, 18, 61, 129, 132, 185, 242
communities, 58, 81, 100, 203, 240
Communities That Care (CTC), 203
community, 10, 11, 17, 22, 50, 51, 60, 61, 82, 83, 87, 104, 117, 138, 141, 144, 200, 202, 227, 236, 240, 248
community service, 11
competition, 12, 143
complement, 134
comprehension, 150
Comprehensive Social Security Assistance, 206
computer, 167
conception, 224
conceptual model, 18
conference, 53, 100, 252, 253
confidentiality, 183, 204
configuration, 184
conflict resolution, 17, 61, 242
consciousness, 148, 155
consent, 183, 204, 248
construction, 116, 162, 176
consumption, 243, 248
content analysis, 139
control group, 6, 7, 34, 47, 50, 58, 61, 62, 63, 65, 66, 67, 68, 69, 70, 71, 72, 74, 75, 78, 79, 80, 88, 139, 144, 145, 161
controlled trials, 22, 80
controversial, 48
convergence, 90, 175
cooperation, 126, 144
coordination, 148, 149
correlation, 106, 186, 202, 205, 206, 207, 216, 217
cost, xx, 50, 133, 243, 244, 248
cough, 180, 185, 189, 206, 213, 244, 252, 253
counseling, 61, 62, 104, 112, 144, 252
crimes, 14

critical thinking, 17
cultivation, 104, 121, 124
cultural beliefs, 14
cultural conditions, 193
culture, 4, 28, 48, 86, 99, 105, 162, 180, 234, 241, 243, 244, 245, 247, 271
cure, 138
curriculum, 17, 18, 20, 181, 241, 244

D

dance, 61, 272
DAT deterrent effects, 49
data analysis, 44, 136, 140, 157, 270
data collection, 44, 50, 115, 121, 140, 155, 156, 183, 204, 205, 208, 210
database, 203
deduction, 15
delinquency, 14, 15, 23, 65, 80, 182, 192, 196, 197, 225, 227, 245
delinquent behavior, 58, 83, 120, 228
demand characteristic, 115, 156, 175
demographic characteristics, 210
demographic factors, 209
Denmark, 266
Department of Education, 30, 52, 265
Department of Health and Human Services, 53, 193, 195
dependent variable, 67, 139, 208, 209, 217, 218, 219, 220, 222
depressants, 180
depressive symptoms, 229
depth, 21, 31, 37, 38, 43, 62, 115, 120, 121, 134, 135, 139, 140, 152, 154, 155, 224
detection, 29, 37
detention, 32
deterrence, 53
developmental change, 196
developmental psychopathology, 82, 135
deviation, 216
directors, 32
disability, 258, 264, 266
disclosure, 50
diseases, 143
distortions, 16
distress, 229
distribution, 63, 197
diversity, 134, 139, 155
divorce rates, 242
dosage, 150
drinking patterns, 197
drug abuse, 5, 28, 36, 53, 58, 79, 81, 82, 86, 100, 105, 121, 123, 124, 126, 131, 132, 135, 142, 147, 149, 150, 154, 156, 181, 191, 200, 201, 202, 203, 208, 209, 235, 236, 237, 238, 240, 245, 252
drug abusers, 132, 202, 237
drug addict, xxi, 104, 105, 166, 172, 173, 175, 248
drug addiction, xxi, 105, 248
drug education, 8, 23, 37, 51, 82, 83, 87, 246, 247, 249
drug resistance, 23
drug testing, xiii, 7, 27, 28, 29, 31, 32, 33, 34, 35, 36, 37, 38, 39, 40, 41, 42, 45, 46, 48, 49, 50, 51, 52, 53, 83, 100, 117, 156, 177
drug treatment, 104

E

eating disorders, 271
ecology, 227
economic disadvantage, 82, 83
economic status, 202, 204, 206, 209, 223
ecstasy, xx, 4, 60, 64, 68, 69, 71, 72, 78, 180, 185, 186, 206, 210, 214, 215
editors, xi, xiv, 257
education, 8, 10, 11, 23, 37, 38, 51, 81, 82, 83, 87, 89, 105, 162, 177, 203, 224, 236, 246, 247, 248, 249, 261, 272
educational programs, 104, 105
educational settings, 177, 178
educators, 53
elementary school, 203
emotion, 12, 14, 131
emotional distress, 229
emotional reactions, 17
empathy, 15, 17

empirical studies, 29, 48
employment, 224
encouragement, 132
endurance, 16
enforcement, 42, 236, 248
England, xx
environment, 58, 120, 193, 240, 249
environmental factors, 59, 121
environmental influences, 59, 121
epidemic, 201
evidence, xiii, 7, 8, 9, 10, 13, 15, 16, 22, 23, 25, 45, 48, 49, 51, 54, 58, 59, 68, 70, 72, 78, 79, 80, 81, 82, 99, 105, 106, 116, 117, 130, 155, 157, 160, 176, 177, 224, 226, 249, 251
evidence-based program, 8, 22
experimental condition, 81
experimental design, 6, 49, 62, 139
exposure, 12, 182, 192, 223
expulsion, 32
extraneous variable, 6

F

facilitators, 109
FAI, 185, 195
fairness, 35, 40, 46, 52
faith, 240
families, 20, 82, 86, 131, 151, 183, 192, 194, 202, 204, 220, 223, 229, 240, 241, 242, 243, 248, 249, 251, 253
Family Assessment Instrument, 185, 190, 195
family characteristics, 205, 206, 209
family environment, 58, 120, 249
family factors, 180, 204, 208, 210, 217, 219, 220, 221, 223, 226, 241, 245
family functioning, 180, 185, 186, 187, 188, 189, 190, 194, 195
family life, 204, 206, 209, 217, 220, 224, 247
family members, 88, 93, 122, 129, 185
family relationships, 60, 192
family system, 246
family therapy, 136, 157
feelings, 17, 38, 123, 125, 129, 141, 151
financial, 184, 186, 200

Finland, 265
fitness, 144
focus groups, 136, 156, 157
football, 10
force, 5, 234, 235, 236
Ford, 10, 23
formation, 18, 104, 114
foundations, 10, 11, 12, 13, 22
friendship, 87, 138
funding, 10, 11, 12, 13, 22
funds, 11, 12

G

gambling, 11, 23, 191, 244, 247, 253
gender differences, 20
generalizability, 176
Germany, xx, 266
gerontology, 264
goal setting, 17
grades, 39
grants, 11
graph, 172, 174
grids, 165
group activities, 91, 95, 112, 126, 146, 147, 148
group work, 94, 146, 148, 152, 154
growth, 173, 197, 228, 241
guidance, xxi, 241
guidelines, 246, 248

H

happiness, xix, xx
harmful effects, 23, 124, 126, 133
harmony, 185, 253
hazards, 240
health, xix, xx, 11, 16, 19, 28, 53, 65, 89, 117, 133, 180, 181, 192, 193, 195, 196, 200, 203, 227, 236, 243, 248, 258, 264, 266, 269, 270, 271, 272
Health and Human Services, 53, 193, 195
health care, 271
health effects, 270
health problems, 16, 133, 243, 248

Index

health services, 117
heroin, xx, 64, 68, 69, 70, 72, 78, 160, 189, 206, 210, 214, 215, 222
high school, 6, 14, 28, 32, 33, 34, 35, 36, 38, 39, 40, 41, 42, 50, 52, 65, 195
history, 99, 106, 248
HIV, 194
holistic care, 162
holistic medicine, 271
holistic psychiatric rehabilitation, 162, 164, 177
homes, 5, 197, 235
homicide, 200
House, 53, 265
human, xix, xx, xxi, 13, 22, 89, 99, 106, 135, 157, 193, 227, 258, 264, 266, 269
human development, 227, 258, 264, 266, 269
human rights, 194
husband, 242, 243, 247
hypothesis, 139, 223
hypothesis test, 139

I

Iceland, 201
ideal, 136, 157, 163, 166, 172, 173, 175, 176, 253
identification, 18, 31, 122, 142, 164, 167, 181, 191, 192, 200, 248
identity, 18, 62, 115, 160, 162, 163, 164, 172, 175, 177, 182, 184, 188, 189, 191, 203, 209, 221, 224, 225
illicit drug use, 4, 28, 32, 33, 38, 39, 52, 53, 180, 181, 189, 201, 202, 225, 234
image, 87, 148
immigration, 246, 248
implicit association test, 226
improvements, 38, 132
impulses, 17
income, 36, 41, 51, 224
incompatibility, 59, 120
independence, 126
independent variable, 176, 209
indirect measure, 226

individual character, 220
individuals, 120, 162, 182, 191, 192, 193
induction, 15
information processing, 228
ingredients, 112, 126
initiation, 194, 225, 228
injuries, 200
inner world, 156
inoculation, 245, 249
integration, 6, 22, 270
integrity, 15
interaction effects, 79
intercourse, 127, 128
internal consistency, 46
International Narcotics Control, 4, 28, 234
interpersonal skills, 17, 126, 151, 242
intervention, 7, 10, 13, 15, 19, 22, 34, 39, 59, 65, 71, 79, 83, 116, 160, 176, 201, 203, 228, 240, 249, 250, 251
intervention strategies, 201, 240
Israel, xiv, 4, 258, 263, 264, 266, 267, 272
issues, 15, 16, 19, 20, 24, 28, 29, 49, 51, 117, 127, 252

J

juvenile delinquency, 15, 23

K

kindergarten, 228
knowledge acquisition, 104, 153

L

labeling, 144
landscape, 135
law enforcement, 42, 236, 248
laws, 15
lead, 16, 142, 202, 226, 236, 251
leadership, 61, 153
learning, xxi, 11, 19, 124, 258
learning difficulties, 11

legal issues, 127
legality, 52
leisure, 194
life satisfaction, 182, 204, 206, 209, 217, 220, 224, 226, 258
lifetime, 138, 201
light, 193, 243, 244, 248
line graph, 172, 174
linear model, 47
local community, 236
longitudinal study, xiv, 58, 62, 82, 83, 120, 183, 196, 199, 203, 204
love, 185, 242

M

Mainland China, 184
majority, 110, 113, 130, 131, 181
management, 17, 60, 98, 271
manipulation, 176
manpower, 144, 249
marijuana, 39, 60, 64, 67, 68, 69, 70, 72, 78
marital status, 184, 186, 204, 206, 209, 210, 217, 218, 220, 223
marriage, 162, 184, 186, 190, 206, 210, 215, 221, 223
materials, 91, 95, 107, 110, 135, 143
matter, xi, 127
measurement, 139, 177, 204, 225
media, 60, 87
medical, 11, 104, 258, 272
medicine, 24, 89, 180, 213, 239, 244, 252, 253, 266, 270, 272
memory, 133
mental disorder, 272
mental health, 16, 19, 117, 195, 227, 243, 248
mental retardation, 12
mentorship, 247
messages, 123, 146, 149, 154
meta-analysis, 23, 197, 252
methodology, 29, 61, 164
Mexico, xx
migration, 271
military, 175
Minneapolis, 228

mission, 264
models, 19, 20, 47, 81, 105, 135, 157, 192, 252
modern society, 116
modifications, 91, 106
mold, 270
Monitoring the Future (MTF), 180
mood disorder, 271
morale, 31, 38, 51
motivation, 20, 258
MSW, 57, 119, 262
multidimensional, 224
multigroup confirmatory factor analyses (MCFA), 184, 185
multiple regression, 187, 209
multiple regression analyses, 187
multiple regression analysis, 209
multivariate statistics, 83
mutuality, 185, 189
mycotoxins, 270

N

narcotics, 236
narratives, 131, 139, 153
National Household Survey on Drug Abuse (NHSDA), 28, 180
National Survey, 28, 180, 195
needy, 10, 12, 13, 249
negative experiences, 134, 145, 242
neglect, 270
neutral, 125, 130, 206, 208
New Zealand, 117
next generation, 266
Nobel Prize, 258
North America, 180, 182, 191
Norway, 266

O

obstacles, xvii, 7, 22, 145
offenders, 167, 178, 227
officials, 15
old age, 220
Opium Wars, xx

Index

opportunities, 17, 20, 150, 196, 242, 244
optimism, 240
ownership, 250

P

P.A.T.H.S., 8, 10, 11, 16, 22, 23, 24, 25, 54, 100, 101, 117, 134, 136, 157, 177, 193, 197, 203, 204, 224, 226, 227, 228
Pacific, 100, 117, 253, 266
pain, 270
paradigm shift, 23
parental consent, 248
parental involvement, 20, 120
parental support, 241
parenting, 58, 121, 182, 185, 226, 242, 247, 249, 253
parents, 5, 35, 37, 46, 60, 82, 129, 136, 145, 147, 149, 157, 173, 186, 196, 206, 221, 223, 235, 242, 243, 244, 247, 249, 253
pathology, 160
peer group, 196
peer influence, 58, 60, 127, 180, 192, 235, 241, 242, 246
peer relationship, 240
permit, 6, 14, 156, 175, 176
personal development, 93, 109, 202, 244
personal problems, 250
personal views, 93
personality, 162
physical laws, 15
pilot study, 52
planning decisions, 140
playing, 115, 132, 153
PM, 52, 53, 193
PMS, 215, 216, 218, 219, 220, 221, 222
police, 5, 62, 235, 249
policy, 4, 5, 11, 23, 24, 28, 35, 40, 46, 48, 49, 52, 53, 80, 180, 246, 247, 248, 249, 251, 261, 266
politics, 12, 197
population, 48, 195, 209, 223, 243, 244, 247, 249
positive attitudes, 123, 142

positive reinforcement, 109
positive youth development (PYD), 181
poverty, 12, 15, 202, 223
pragmatism, 6
PRC, 3, 9, 11, 27, 57, 85, 103, 119, 137, 159, 179, 199, 233, 234, 235, 257, 258, 261, 263, 269
preparation, xi, 23, 51, 227, 251
primary function, 122, 142
principles, 6, 12, 19, 20, 24, 50, 121, 139, 155
prisons, 14
probability, 218, 220
problem behavior, 81, 83, 138, 181, 182, 191, 192, 193, 194, 195, 196, 197, 203, 224, 225, 226, 228
problem behaviors, 191, 192, 193, 195, 203, 224
problem-solving, 17
professionals, 5, 28, 89, 176, 180, 264, 266
profit, 10
project, 6, 7, 10, 11, 12, 16, 18, 20, 22, 58, 59, 61, 62, 80, 81, 83, 87, 88, 90, 105, 106, 121, 140, 141, 142, 143, 149, 161, 183, 203, 224, 243, 258, 262, 266
Project Astro MIND, 82, 86, 88, 100, 116, 141, 157, 161, 162, 177
Project D.A.R.E. (Drug Abuse Resistance Education), 6, 14
proliferation, 81, 105
prosocial behavior, 18
protection, 229, 248
protective factors, 5, 58, 81, 82, 88, 104, 116, 121, 135, 161, 181, 182, 192, 194, 201, 203, 218, 220, 221, 222, 226, 245, 251
psychiatric patients, 116
psychiatry, 271
psychological development, 193, 196
psychological health, 65, 258
psychological well-being, 31, 38, 65, 81, 83, 88, 161, 181, 194, 195
psychology, 89, 159, 162, 177, 194, 195, 258, 271
psychometric properties, 117
psychopathology, 82, 135, 196

psychopharmacology, xxi, 272
psychotherapy, 117, 162
psychotropic drugs, 60, 63, 64, 69, 71, 72, 73, 86, 215, 222, 234, 235, 244
puberty, 87, 138, 225
public concern, 48
public health, 181, 264, 266, 270, 271
public service, 264
punishment, 14, 243, 244, 248

Q

qualitative research, 53, 121, 135, 139, 140, 157
quality of life, 228, 258, 271
quantitative research, 49
query, 156
questionnaire, 62, 63, 116, 117, 148, 150, 176, 183, 205, 208

R

race, 10
random assignment, 6
rating scale, 89, 163, 164
reactions, 17
reality, 162
recreational, 11, 191, 194
recruiting, 132, 144, 145, 204
Registry, 4, 86, 192, 196, 201, 234, 235, 237, 238
regression, 187, 208, 209, 210, 217, 220, 225
regression analysis, 209, 220
regression model, 209
rehabilitation program, 177
reinforcement, 18, 109
relevance, 24, 177, 252
reliability, 15, 51, 65, 66, 92, 93, 94, 97, 98, 99, 100, 109, 110, 112, 113, 115, 121, 123, 124, 125, 126, 129, 130, 132, 133, 134, 140, 142, 146, 147, 148, 149, 152, 153, 155, 156, 185
researchers, 6, 50, 65, 87, 121, 123, 134, 138, 140, 143, 155, 156, 175, 176, 203, 236, 269

resilience, 181, 184, 188, 189, 203, 229, 240, 252
resistance, 17, 23, 104, 114, 125, 133, 145
resolution, 17, 61, 242
resources, xxi, 104, 106, 144, 156, 175, 182, 202, 250, 251
response, 5, 18, 116, 117, 145, 155, 161, 185, 190, 193
restoration, 104
retardation, 12
risk, xiii, 5, 14, 39, 41, 57, 58, 59, 81, 82, 87, 88, 104, 120, 121, 138, 161, 181, 182, 191, 192, 195, 196, 200, 201, 202, 203, 218, 220, 222, 223, 224, 225, 226, 229, 234, 236, 240, 241, 244, 246, 248, 249, 251
roots, 270
Rosenberg Self-Esteem Scale, 65
routines, 142
rowing, 202
rules, 18, 123, 153

S

scarcity, 190
school activities, 29, 242, 246
school adjustment, 81, 83, 194, 195
school improvement, 20
school performance, 58, 120, 151, 200, 203, 204, 206, 226
science, 13, 15, 83, 241, 264
scope, 223
search terms, 29
secondary data, 100
secondary school students, 53, 90, 138, 200, 203, 226
secondary schools, 5, 60, 201, 204
secondary students, 191, 201
security assistance, 186, 190
self-confidence, 128, 173
self-control, 171
self-discipline, 153
self-efficacy, 18, 20, 184, 188, 189, 240
self-esteem, 58, 60, 65, 113, 120, 229
self-identity, 62, 160, 162, 163, 164, 172, 175, 177, 182, 203

self-image, 87, 148
self-knowledge, 128
self-reflection, 20, 147, 150
self-regulation, 196
self-understanding, 60, 87, 151
sellers, 244
sensation, 120, 240
sensation seeking, 240
sensitivity, 50, 61
sentencing, 246, 248
services, xi, 11, 13, 61, 89, 98, 99, 100, 106, 117, 134, 135, 143, 157, 241, 245, 246, 249, 250, 251
sex, 19, 59, 60, 64, 65, 67, 68, 69, 72, 78, 79, 87, 88, 91, 94, 96, 97, 107, 108, 109, 111, 112, 114, 122, 125, 127, 128, 130, 131, 142, 147, 148, 151, 152, 153, 154, 161
sexual activities, 139
sexual activity, 191
sexual behavior, 64, 65, 72, 78, 90, 196
sexual intercourse, 127, 128
sexuality, 271
showing, 6, 14, 48, 78, 79, 99, 106, 171, 182, 225, 240, 241, 243, 245
siblings, 242, 246
silver, 50
skills training, 58, 105, 153
smoking, 59, 64, 67, 68, 69, 70, 72, 78, 87, 90, 91, 93, 94, 96, 97, 107, 108, 111, 114, 124, 151, 185, 191, 201, 210, 222, 225
social behavior, 63, 202
social capital, 245
social competence, 58, 121, 184, 188, 189, 191, 196, 203, 224
social costs, 160
social information processing, 228
social justice, 18
social policy, 261
social problems, 12, 235
social resources, 104
social responsibility, 10
social sciences, 83, 135
social security, 186, 190
Social Security, 206

social skills, 58, 63, 68, 72, 78, 79, 86, 88, 91, 92, 94, 96, 97, 105, 107, 108, 110, 111, 112, 114, 120, 161
social stress, 241
social workers, xiii, 19, 60, 62, 81, 103, 104, 105, 106, 107, 108, 110, 112, 114, 115, 134, 138, 249, 261
society, 10, 12, 104, 105, 116, 201, 225, 236, 264
solidarity, 16, 243, 247
solution, 28
spastic, 61
spending, 19
spirituality, 184, 188, 189
SSA, 206
stakeholders, 176, 250, 251
standard deviation, 216, 217
states, 13, 235
statistics, 43, 44, 45, 47, 83, 139, 180, 210, 215, 217, 253
stress, 60, 88, 93, 98, 112, 125, 128, 161, 225, 229, 240, 241, 252
stressful events, 17
structure, 20, 192, 194, 197
structuring, 140
style, 104, 105, 240
subgroups, 185
subjective experience, 88, 89, 134, 140, 156
substance use, xiv, 49, 116, 135, 180, 181, 182, 185, 186, 187, 188, 189, 190, 191, 192, 193, 194, 195, 196, 200, 201, 202, 203, 208, 210, 216, 217, 218, 220, 222, 223, 224, 225, 226, 227, 228, 229
success rate, 160
suicidal ideation, 258
suicide, 16, 271
Sun, ix, xi, xiii, xiv, xxi, 8, 10, 24, 54, 100, 136, 157, 194, 228, 229, 258
supervision, 223, 243, 247
supervisors, 262
Supreme Court, 28, 49
surplus, 11
surveillance, 195
sustainability, 49

Sweden, 266
symptoms, 117, 229
syndrome, 242, 243, 247
synthesis, 228

T

tactics, 250
Tai Po district, 48
Taiwan, 252
target, 58, 109, 120, 223
teacher training, 203
teachers, 19, 21, 62, 128, 133, 150, 151
teaching strategies, 19
team members, 144
teams, 31, 37, 38
technology, 13, 178
teens, 68, 69, 70, 80
territory, 195
test data, 167
testing program, 31, 32, 33, 34, 35, 36, 37, 38, 39, 40, 41, 44, 52, 53
textbook, 271
therapy, 136, 157, 177, 270
thoughts, 127, 160, 162, 244
time frame, 13, 64, 66, 245
tobacco, 185, 191, 196, 200, 201, 202, 206, 210, 222, 225
trainees, 20
training, 11, 19, 20, 21, 58, 61, 90, 101, 104, 105, 106, 121, 124, 141, 143, 144, 153, 157, 203, 261
training programs, 20, 101
trajectory, 222, 240
tranquilizers, 4, 86, 180, 234
treatment, 6, 37, 50, 104, 117, 139, 160, 236, 250, 271
trial, 21, 48, 52, 53, 83, 176, 228
triangulation, 6, 21, 51, 62, 90, 114, 123, 134, 143, 155, 175

U

United Nations, 4, 28, 194, 201, 234
United States, xix, xx, 4, 24, 28, 52, 105, 194, 195, 201, 228, 234, 253, 258
universities, 16
USA, 31, 32, 33, 34, 35, 36, 37, 38, 39, 40, 41, 42, 257

V

validation, 116, 117, 194
valuation, 91, 95, 107, 110, 116, 135, 157, 228
variables, 6, 65, 67, 120, 139, 187, 192, 193, 209, 210, 215, 216, 217, 218, 220, 222
vein, 58
venue, 98, 148
videos, 150
violence, 6, 14, 16, 19, 192, 196
vulnerability, 59, 82, 121, 135

W

Washington, 35, 53, 82, 135
welfare programs, 22
well-being, 31, 38, 51, 65, 81, 83, 88, 161, 181, 194, 195, 258
work activities, 94
workers, 4, 7, 19, 20, 24, 60, 61, 62, 81, 86, 88, 92, 94, 95, 99, 104, 105, 106, 107, 108, 110, 111, 112, 114, 115, 124, 132, 133, 134, 137, 138, 140, 142, 143, 144, 145, 148, 149, 152, 153, 154, 155, 161, 236, 249, 261

Y

young adults, xx, 196

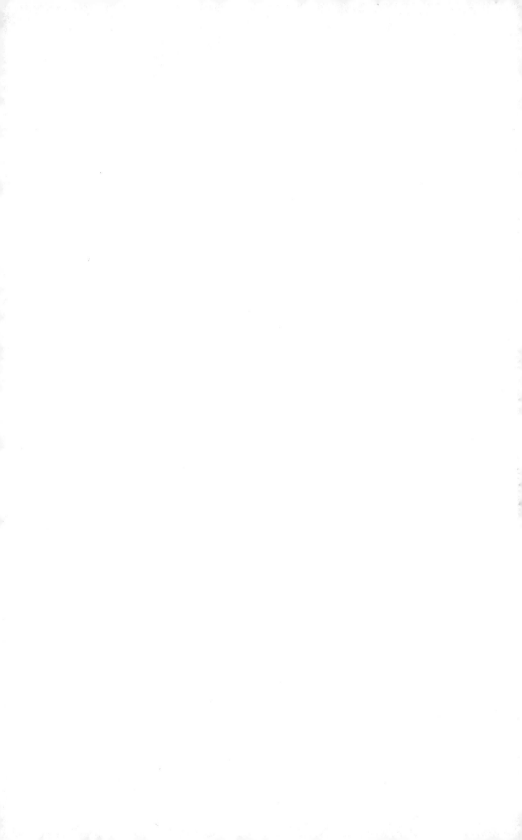